**This book is to be returned on or before
the last date stamped below.**

Posterior Uveitis:
Diagnosis and Management

Posterior Uveitis: Diagnosis and Management

KHALID F. TABBARA, M.D.

Professor and Chairman
Department of Ophthalmology
College of Medicine
King Saud University
Riyadh, Saudi Arabia

ROBERT B. NUSSENBLATT, M.D.

Clinical Director
National Eye Institute
Bethesda, Maryland

Foreword by Ronald E. Smith, M.D.

Professor and Chairman
University of Southern California
School of Medicine
Department of Opthalmology
Immediate Past President
American Uveitis Society

Butterworth–Heinemann
Boston   London   Oxford   Singapore   Sydney   Toronto   Wellington

Every effort has been made to ensure that the drug dosage schedules within this text are accurate and conform to standards accepted at time of publication. However, as treatment recommendations vary in the light of continuing research and clinical experience, the reader is advised to verify drug dosage schedules herein with information found on product information sheets. This is especially true in cases of new or infrequently used drugs.

 Recognizing the importance of preserving what has been written, it is the policy of Butterworth–Heinemann to have the books it publishes printed on acid-free paper, and we exert our best efforts to that end.

Library of Congress Cataloging-in-Publication Data
Tabbara, Khalid F.
    Posterior Uveitis : diagnosis and management / Khalid F. Tabbara,
Robert B. Nussenblatt.
        p.   cm.
    Includes bibliographical references and index.
    ISBN 0-7506-9599-4 (alk. paper : hardcover)
    1. Posterior uveitis.   I. Nussenblatt, Robert B.   II. Title.
    [DNLM   1. Uveitis. Posterior—diagnosis.   2. Uveitis, Posterior—
therapy.   WW 240 T112p 1994]
RE353.T33   1994
617.7'2—dc20
DNLM/DLC
for Library of Congress   94-32315
                                                               CIP

British Library Cataloguing-in-Publication Data
A catalogue record for this book is available from the British Library.

Butterworth–Heinemann
313 Washington Street
Newton, MA 02158-1626

10 9 8 7 6 5 4 3 2 1

Printed in the United States of America

To our wives, Najwa and Rosine

Contents

III / NONINFECTIOUS DISEASES

Foreword

Uveitis remains an important cause of ocular morbidity and visual disability. In fact, 10% of visual impairment in the United States is secondary to uveitis. A recent increase in the HIV infected individuals has contributed to an increase in the immunocompromised host population setting the stage for a wide variety of opportunistic infections that afflict the ocular structures.

Arriving at a correct diagnosis in patients with posterior uveitis is a major challenge to every clinician and a decisive opportunity in the outcome of the disease. Early diagnosis and prompt treatment are mandatory for visual rehabilitation and for the prevention of the sequence of posterior uveitis.

This book by Dr. Tabbara and Dr. Nussenblatt presents the complex subject of posterior uveitis in a lucid and succinct manner. The book focuses on the clinical and ocular manifestations of disorders affecting the posterior segment of the eye and elaborates on the current methods of therapy. The clinical findings described in each section are reinforced by colored photographs of the condition. This illustrative display is crucial in the clinical diagnosis. The book provides authoritative information regarding diagnosis and management of various inflammatory conditions affecting the posterior segment. The authors are teachers in the field of uveitis and have contributed to the literature through basic and clinical studies in uveitis. Dr. Tabbara and Dr. Nussenblatt have also presented courses on posterior uveitis for the past 15 years at the Annual Meetings of the American Academy of Ophthalmology.

From my perspective as a worker in the field of uveitis, I believe that this book is a major asset for the clinician and an excellent update of our knowledge in uveitis. The emergence of new opportunistic infections and the resurgence of old diseases make this book invaluable. It is to the credit of the authors who responded to the need in a well-illustrated book on posterior uveitis. We are grateful for their efforts.

Ronald E. Smith, M.D.

Preface

Inflammatory disorders of the uvea can be classified into (1) anterior uveitis, (2) intermediate uveitis, and (3) posterior uveitis. Uveitis may be unilateral or bilateral. There are many entities that lead to posterior uveitis, including infections, autoimmune disorders, malignant diseases, and disorders of unknown origin.

Posterior uveitis is a common cause of ocular morbidity and may lead to visual loss. The most frequently encountered causes of posterior uveitis include Behcet's disease, Vogt-Koyanagi-Harada, and toxoplasmosis. Although most lesions that are designated posterior uveitis can be attributed to some form of infection, others may be regarded as a form of immunologically mediated disease triggered by exogenous factors and endogenous susceptibility. The main objectives of this book are (1) to define and to elucidate the diagnostic signs and laboratory workup of certain common entities of posterior uveitis, and (2) to discuss the differential diagnosis and management of posterior uveitis. The book is also concerned with the systematic scrutiny of the clinical signs and symptoms and the tailored laboratory investigation necessary to arrive at the correct clinical diagnosis in patients presenting with posterior uveitis. The treatment of each entity is outlined at the end of each section.

The therapeutic strategy in uveitis is evolving at a rapid pace. Our improved understanding of the pathogenesis of uveitis is a reflection of the recent advances in the field of immunology, genetics, and molecular biology. Researchers in the field of uveitis are working in concert to dispel the mystery of uveitis, to replace speculations with facts, and to help provide a rational classification of the disorders affecting the uvea. This book provides a concise approach for the diagnosis and management of posterior uveitis.

We wish to acknowledge the editorial assistance of Paula Fedeski-Koundakjian and the outstanding efforts of Susan Pioli of Butterworth-Heinemann.

Khalid F. Tabbara, M.D.
Robert B. Nussenblatt, M.D.

I
Grading of Uveitis

Chapter 1
Introduction

Khalid F. Tabbara

The diagnosis of posterior uveitis can be established in most cases on the basis of (1) the morphology of the lesions, (2) the mode of onset and course of the disease, and (3) the association with other systemic diseases. Laboratory tests are of use mainly in the refinement of the diagnosis or in the elimination of certain diagnoses that might otherwise need to be considered.

From the point of view of morphology, lesions of the posterior segment can be considered to be focal, geographic, or diffuse. Those that cause clouding of the overlying vitreous must be differentiated from those that never cause vitreous clouding. Lesions that are regularly associated with retinal vasculitis, juxtapapillary disease, or serous detachments of the retina must be separately designated. The type and distribution of vitreous opacities must be stipulated.

Inflammatory lesions of the posterior segment are generally insidious in their onset, but some may be accompanied by the abrupt development of vitreous clouding and visual loss. As a general rule, such diseases are also accompanied by anterior uveitis, which, in turn, is sometimes associated with secondary glaucoma.

Many cases of posterior uveitis are associated with some form of systemic disease. Two major categories of systemic disease must be distinguished at the outset: infectious and noninfectious. Although most lesions that are designated "posterior uveitis" can be attributed to some form of infection, others have not been assigned a noninfectious origin. Conspicuous examples of this include Behcet's disease and sarcoidosis. Ultimately, the technique of chorioretinal biopsy may permit infectious agents to be isolated from these lesions, but until such time as that becomes possible, other disease mechanisms must be considered.

Each of the known entities in posterior uveitis (i.e., those that have been confirmed by histopathologic studies or by isolations of organisms) has a rather characteristic picture. Ocular toxoplasmosis, for example, is a focal necrotizing retinochoroiditis that is insidious in onset. The active lesion is generally seen in the company of old, healed scars that may be heavily pigmented. The lesions may be juxtapapillary in location and often give rise to retinal vasculitis. The vitreous is generally very extensively clouded. Such patients usually show no signs of systemic disease, but the toxoplasma dye test is always positive, even though the titer of antibodies may be very low.

By contrast, the lesions of the "presumed ocular histoplasmosis syndrome" consist of multiple tiny choroidal foci that never cloud the overlying vitreous. There is often evidence of peripapillary scarring. The macular lesions of the presumed ocular histoplasmosis syndrome may produce subretinal neovascular nets. Bleeding from these nets is common, and this produces a "signet ring" lesion that is bluish or bluish-gray in color. There are generally no signs of systemic disease, although an x-ray of the chest may show evidence of disseminated calcific foci in the peripheral portions of the lung fields, and an x-ray of the abdomen may show no evidence of antihistoplasma antibodies, but an intradermal skin test will show evidence of delayed hypersensitivity responses to histoplasmin in more than 85% of the cases.

The lesions of cytomegalic inclusion disease produce geographic infiltrates in the retina, often accompanied by occlusive retinal vasculitis and hemorrhage. Such lesions rarely produce vitreous clouding in adult cases, whereas neonatal cases may be characterized by a very cloudy vitreous. In adults cytomegalic inclusion disease of the retina is seen almost exclusively among immunologically compromised hosts. Patients who are receiving cytotoxic immunosuppressive agents to retard the rejection of an organ transplant and AIDS patients are prime examples of individuals who might suffer from this kind of retinal disease. They also may develop encephalitis from the same infection, but often they are free of other systemic complaints. Cytomegalic inclusions often can be recovered from their urine, and the serum may show the presence of antibodies that can be detected by a complement fixation test or by an enzyme-linked immunosorbent assay (ELISA) test.

These are only a few examples of the types of analysis that can be applied to the differential diagnosis of posterior uveitis. The examiner is required to learn the basic clinical characteristic of each disease, but success in diagnosing most posterior inflammations of the choroid and retina will result from application of these principles.

Chapter 2

Grading of Intermediate and Posterior Uveitis

John V. Forrester, David BenEzra, Robert B. Nussenblatt, Khalid F. Tabbara, and Penti Timonen

Advances in our understanding of the pathogenic mechanisms involved in uveitis and uveoretinitis led to the introduction of various new therapeutic modalities for these diseases.[1] Studies regarding the effectiveness of these therapies in endogenous uveitis have been equivocal and disappointing.[2,3] This situation has led to the search for newer and potent modalities.[4–6] It was soon realized, however, that assessment of drug efficacy based solely on visual acuity is insufficient and does not reflect properly the entire spectrum of disease manifestations. Therefore, the need for a complete, thorough, and reproducible standard scoring system was raised during the analysis of a masked study evaluating the effectiveness of cyclosporin A (CsA) versus conventional therapy in Behcet's disease.[7] This was followed by the formation of a study group whose task was to prepare a universal grading system that would reflect both the intraocular inflammatory activity and the visual acuity and could be used as a standard system throughout the world.

This monograph is the end result of extensive consultations and discussions carried out during the years 1988 through 1990. The Hogan-Kimura-Thygeson system suggested during the 1950s is based on slit-lamp examination and the macroscopic appearance of the anterior segment.[8] This system was introduced during the early days of increasing use of the slit lamp. It emphasizes the degree of cellular infiltrate and protein exudate in the aqueous humor.

These authors also developed their system to include the posterior segment, particularly by grading the degree of vitreous opacity as seen through the direct ophthalmoscope.[9] Although adopted by most practicing ophthalmologists, it soon became evident that this system has many limitations:

1. A recognized standard for each grade of uveitis has not been fully established.
2. There exists some confusion concerning the relative importance of other associated manifestations of the anterior segment such as iris vessel dilatation, keratic precipitates (KPs), synechiae, iris nodules, iris atrophy, and band keratopathy. Some of these signs are sequelae to the uveitis state and may not represent active disease.
3. Considerable importance has been placed on the precise description of the KP as to whether a uveitis is granulomatous or nongranulomatous. Experience and follow-up observations have shown that a uveitis may start as "nongranulomatous" and show "granulomatous" manifestations later or vice versa.
4. A great variability in grading the posterior segment manifestations was obtained when the observations were made by different observers.
5. The use of the direct ophthalmoscope and the corneal contact lens as suggested by Hogan, Kimura, and Thygeson for evaluation of the posterior segment inflammation did not permit the evaluation and comparison of the degree of

vitreous opacity observed during various visits. Also, it is difficult to properly evaluate the extent of vitreous haze observed with a direct ophthalmoscope when the examination is performed through a widely dilated pupil and a clear lens, or when examination is carried out through a poorly dilated pupil (presence of posterior synechiae) with some degree of posterior subcapsular lens opacity.

Nussenblatt et al.[10] took advantage of the fact that the funduscopic view through an indirect ophthalmoscope is less affected by lens opacities and irregular pupils. These authors developed a series of standard photographs that represent various grades of vitreous haze. Despite its apparent vulnerability to observer error, in practice this binocular indirect ophthalmoscopic (BIO) grading of vitreal "haze" has been found to be relatively reliable and reproducible. Still, the proper assessment of the intraocular inflammation of the choroid and retina was lacking. Therefore, an overall evaluation of the disease activity was needed.

The main problem with regard to posterior segment inflammation is the wide range of clinical disorders grouped together under the terms "endogenous uveitis" or chronic intraocular inflammation. Hogan et al.[8] originally described the clinical appearance of posterior uveitis and considered periphlebitis to be a rare phenomenon. They failed to recognize the active, hemorrhagic forms of posterior or peripheral retinal vasculitis. Also, it has become evident that fundal findings that previously would have been accepted as the prototype of discrete localized lesions such as toxoplasma choroidoretinitis may be a manifestation of a more general uveoretinal response. Certain disorders with well-defined clinical signs, such as pars planitis, also show considerable clinical overlap with other disorders.

Furthermore, the Dalen-Fuchs nodule, believed to be a pathognomonic clinical sign of sympathetic ophthalmia, is also observed in Vogt-Koyanagi-Harada (VKH) disease and in sarcoid uveoretinitis. It has been shown that a single retinal antigen can induce an entire range of uveoretinal inflammatory signs. Manipulation of the immunization schedule—varying the dose of the antigen, the species and strain, or the state of immunosuppression in the experimental animal—includes intraocular manifestations similar to those observed in patients during the course of various uveitides.[11,12] When grading these disorders, it therefore may be relatively less important to label the disease with a clinical tag than to describe or grade the severity and extent of retinal and choroidal involvement.

Types of Uveitis

Uveitis may be restricted to the anterior segment, involve the anterior segment and anterior vitreous, or be predominantly a manifestation of the posterior segment with or without signs of inflammation within the anterior chamber. Most forms of chronic uveitis are of unknown origin. Even when infectious agents are suspected, the evidence for their involvement in these chronic cases is at best circumstantial.

The most frequent form of uveitis is acute anterior uveitis, which is, in most cases, a self-limited inflammation characterized by circumcorneal injection, ciliary spasm, and cells and flare in the anterior chamber. If the uveitis is extensive and left untreated, synechiae, abnormalities of intraocular pressure (either hypotension or hypertension) keratic precipitates, and hypopyon/fibrin clots in the anterior chamber and angle structures may develop. In general, the posterior segment is not involved, unless the disorder persists and there is secondary infiltration of cells in the vitreous and secondary macular edema ensues. The acute form of the disease shows a strong association with the major histocompatibility complex Class I antigen HLA-B27 and its related conditions such as ankylosing spondylitis and Reiter's disease. In some cases, an infectious cause is suspected through links with bacterial enterocolitis *Yersinia* and klebsiella in combination with the presence of HLA-B27.[13,14]

Less painful or "silent" chronic forms of anterior uveitis also occur in which the protein exudate (flare) is more prominent in the anterior chamber and the cellular component is less marked. In both the acute and chronic forms, grading of ocular inflammation is readily achieved.

Pars planitis (intermediate uveitis) involves predominantly the peripheral retina and vitreous base and characteristically is associated with vitreous inflammatory cell infiltrates (snowballs). During the course of the disease in some cases, extensive peripheral subretinal chorioretinal infiltrates may develop and progress toward the posterior pole of the fundus. Careful examination and fluorescein angiography demonstrate signs of peripheral retinal vasculitis in many cases. Visual loss in these eyes is most frequently attributable to macular edema.

Posterior uveitis may involve primarily the posterior pole and equatorial region of the choroid and retina. Involvement of the pars plana or the anterior segment may be observed early; characteristically, however, these are observed late during the disease course.

Some patients may show concomitant involvement of the anterior, intermediate, and posterior uveal tissues. The cases are generally coined as pan-uveitides.

Specific Clinical Entities

Some of the most common endogenous noninfectious posterior uveitides are listed in Table 2.1. Sympathetic opthalmia is characterized by extensive choroidal infiltrates and thickening of the choroid. The typical subretinal nodule or microgranuloma (Dalen-Fuchs nodule) is most probably a granulomatous formation identical to the choroidal granulomata settling under the pigment epithelium through breaks within the Bruch's membrane.[15] Using immunohistochemical methods, similar nodules formed mainly by reticuloendothelial system (RES)-derived cells are observed in sarcoidosis,[16] Vogt-Koyanagi-Harada's disease,[17] and also in other inflammatory disorders manifesting as diffuse choroiditis.

Fluorescein angiography during the active phase demonstrates hypofluorescent choroidal "spots" in

Table 2.1. Endogenous (Noninfectious) Posterior Uveitis

Examples of Clinical Entities	Examples of Descriptive Forms
Idiopathic retinal vasculitis	Isolated posterior uveitis
Sarcoid retinitis/vasculitis	Panuveitis
Birdshot choriodoretinopathy	Choroiditis: discrete,
Behcet's disease	focal, diffuse,
Vogt-Koyanagi-Harada disease	serpigineous,
Pigment epitheliopathies	geographic
Presumed ocular histoplasmosis	
Sympathetic ophthalmia	
Intermediate uveitis (pars planitis)	

the early phase with late hyperfluorescence.[18] Healed, inactive lesions are overlaid by depigmented retinal pigment epithelium and appear as pigment epithelial defects on fluorescein angiography.

In cases of "intermediate" uveitis (pars planitis), a few snowball granulomata in the equatorial or preequatorial fundus may be sufficient to cause symptoms of floaters.

Retinal vasculitis involving the posterior pole may present as an "idiopathic" disorder or as part of a disease entity such as sarcoidosis, Behcet's disease, multiple sclerosis, or systemic lupus erythematosis. The vasculitis may affect small or large vessels, and occurs usually as a phlebitis with retinal hemorrhages. In Behcet's disease, however, both arteritis and phlebitis occur, with widespread retinal infiltrates and ischemia leading to retinal necrosis.[19] Retinal vasculitis rarely occurs in isolation. Careful examination shows, in many cases, that chorioretinal infiltrates are also present. In addition, vitreous inflammatory cells are almost a prerequisite for the differentiation of retinal vasculitis from other retinal vascular occlusive disorders.[20]

Some forms of endogenous posterior uveitis, such as sympathetic ophthalmia, appear to affect the choroid more than the retina, although the retina is almost always involved to some degree. The hallmark of these diseases is the widespread distribution of subretinal focal infiltrates and patches of retinal pigment epithelial atrophy. In contrast, retinal vasculitis and acute retinal necrosis might appear to be predominantly retinal disorders. In these cases involvement of the choroid becomes apparent during the late phase of the disease. Vitreous cellular infiltration as the principal intraocular manifestation is characteristic of intermediate uveitis (pars planitis), but retinal and choroidal inflammation occur in this condition as well.

Some disorders appear to have a clear infectious cause, such as herpes simplex–induced acute retinal necrosis, cytomegalovirus retinitis, and toxoplasmic choroidoretinitis. In most uveitis syndromes, however, the cause remains presumptive or undetermined, and the most prominent clinical observations are believed to represent the manifestations of autoimmune phenomena.

Immunohistopathological studies have shown that T cells, T-suppressor (CD8+)[21] and T-helper (CD4+) cells, and monocytes[15] predominate in the choroidal nodules observed in sympathetic ophthalmia and sarcoidosis.[16] Kinetic studies of these infiltrates in experimental autoimmune uveitis in the rat suggest that the T-helper/T-suppressor (CD4+/CD8+) ratio varies during the course of the disease and may be a mechanism of downregulation of the inflammatory process.[22] Some interesting studies of choroidal changes have been reported also in Vogt-Koyanagi-Harada disease.[23] In general, the available histologic data have supported the concept of an immunologically mediated process in most forms of posterior uveitis. Despite the difference in clinical presentation, most forms of posterior uveitis have four cardinal features: (1) inflammatory cells or granulomata within the vitreous; (2) focal chorioretinal infiltrates; (3) retinal vasculitis; and (4) macular edema.

In some forms, there may be a greater emphasis on one or more of these features. In others, additional features may be present such as exudative retinal detachment or subretinal and preretinal neovascularization. These manifestations represent the limited spectrum of possible chorioretinal responses to an inflammatory stimulus. Thus, in clinical practice, the primary ocular stimulus is immunologic, which may follow a previous infectious process, or a combination of both.[1]

Based on the previous experience of the authors in attempting to accurately determine disease activity in uveitis and keeping these limitations in mind, a scoring system may be helpful in assessing the therapeutic effects of antiinflammatory and immunomodulating drugs.

The Scoring System

The following uveitis scoring system has three components: the anterior segment component, the vitreous component, and a fundus component. Each of these is graded and scored separately. A cumulative score should be avoided because, in the presence of extensive opacities of the media (e.g., hypopyon uveitis, cataract, extensive vitreal haze), a fundus grading may not be possible. Thus, an unduly low cumulative score may be obtained. In addition, maintaining a distinction between the anterior and posterior inflammatory grades permits the system to be applied equally to anterior segment-restricted uveitis and to posterior segment disease in which there is secondary anterior segment involvement.

Anterior Segment

Pericorneal injection is considered to be an important manifestation of active inflammation and is recorded as absent or present. No attempt is made to determine the degree of injection. Grading of the anterior findings is solely based on the two "active" and rapidly changing signs, that is, the number of cells and the intensity of flare (Table 2.2). Anterior chamber cells are determined using the widest slit beam at 1-mm height with maximal luminance of the Haag-Streit (or equivalent) slit lamp. Pigment cells and red blood cells are ignored. Anterior chamber flare is determined using the same slit beam and luminance. To enhance the use of standard criteria, an artist's impression of these changes within inflamed eyes is provided (Figure 2.1) and is contrasted with representative black and white photographs.

Secondary features such as keratic precipitates, synechiae, iris vessel dilatations and rubeosis, iris nodules, and secondary corneal changes can be noted but do not add to the score. It should be noted that new Flare-cytometric methods are currently under investigation (e.g., Kowa FC 1000) that may provide the user with a more objective assessment of cells and flare.

Vitreous

Vitreous haze is determined by BIO, using a 20-diopter aspheric lens to observe the posterior pole. Inflammatory activity in the vitreous body can range from the greatest amount of activity (5+) to no evidence (0) of vitreous haze (Table 2.3). A 5+ vitreous haze permits no view of fundal details (using the optic nerve head as a reference point). A 4+ vitreous haze permits only a glimpse of the optic nerve head. A 3+ vitreous haze is one in which details of the optic nerve head are visible but cannot be scrutinized. A 2+ vitreous haze permits the observer to see the optic nerve head details but the view of the disc is fuzzy. A 1+ haze permits good visualization of the retinal vessels and optic nerve but focus on the vitreous body demonstrates the presence of cellular infiltrates. A 0 haze permits clear observation and definition of both the optic nerve head and the retinal vessels without any apparent vitreous haze, as expected from a normal vitreous. Description of the clinical appearance is

Table 2.2. Slit-lamp Biomicroscopy Grading of Anterior Chamber Cells and Flare*

	Cells		Flare
Score	Description	Score	Description
0	Nil: < 5 cells/field	0	Nil to trace
1	Mild: 5–10 cells/field	1	Mild: definitely detectable
2	Moderate: 11–20 cells/field	2	Moderate: without plastic aqueous
3	Marked: 21–50 cells/field	3	Marked: with plastic aqueous
4	Severe: > 50 cells/field	4	Severe: with fibrin deposits or clots
5	Hypopyon formation		

*Field: biomicroscope narrowest slit beam 8 mm in length.

Figure 2.1. Biomicroscopic photographs and artist's drawings showing flare of Grades 0 to 4.

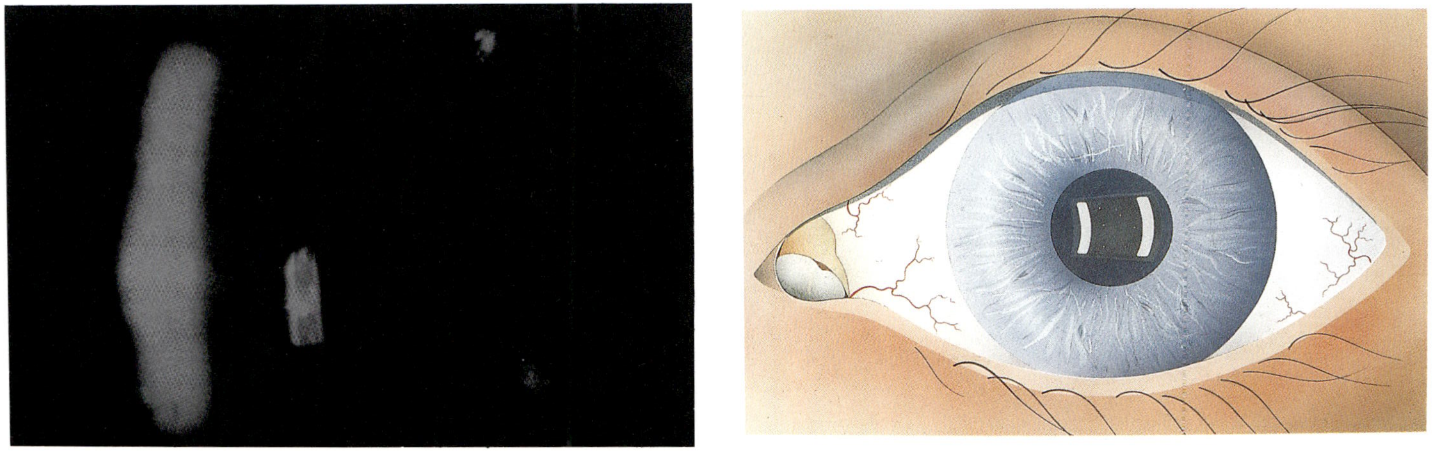

FLARE OF GRADE 0

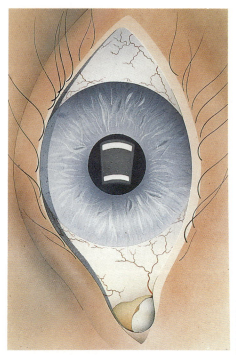

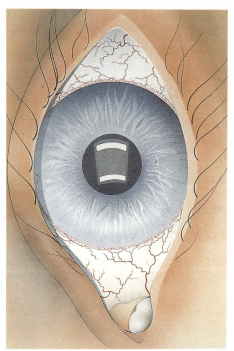

FLARE OF GRADE 1

FLARE OF GRADE 2

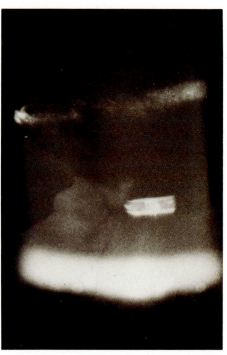

Figure 2.1. (con't.)

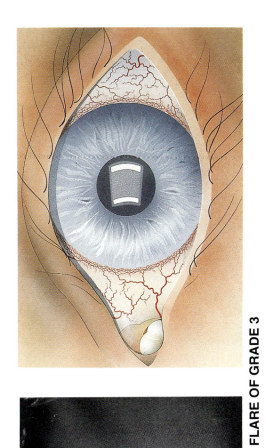

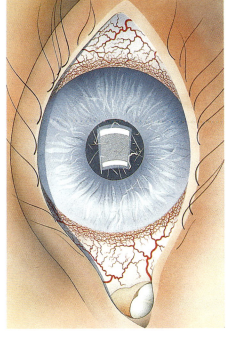

FLARE OF GRADE 3

FLARE OF GRADE 4

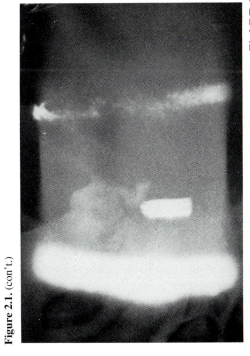

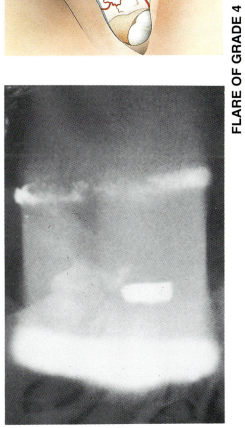

Figure 2.1. (con't.)

provided in Table 2.3, and a comparative series of clinical photographs is available. One should always bear in mind that this assessment may be limited by the presence of lenticular or corneal opacities, hypotony, and recurrent vitreal hemorrhage. In these cases, grading may be markedly influenced by the subjective criteria of the observer. Therefore, in these cases, assessment by two independent ophthalmologists is recommended.

Fundus

For the purposes of grading, the fundus is diagrammatically divided into four pre-equatorial and four postequatorial quadrants (Figure 2.2). Three discrete types of pathology are recognized—retinal vasculitis, chorioretinal infiltrates (lesions), and neovascularization—and the presence of each type of pathology is recorded for each quadrant by marking the appropriate box on the diagram (Figure 2.3).

Retinal Vasculitis

Signs of retinal vasculitis are based solely on activity; in other words, healed lesions are not scored. Indications of activity would include the following: venous engorgement with caliber changes caused by perivascular cuffing with lymphoid infiltrates; hemorrhages accompanying phlebitis; and progressive vascular occlusion, venous or arterial, following sheathing of the vessels with or without cotton wool spots.

Chorioretinal Lesions

Only active inflammatory infiltrates in the choroid and retina are recorded. Signs of activity include

Table 2.3. Grading of Vitreous Haze as Viewed through Binocular Indirect Ophthalmoscope

Score	Description	Clinical Findings
0	Nil	None
1	Minimal	Posterior pole clearly visible
2	Mild	Posterior pole details slightly hazy
3	Moderate	Posterior pole details very hazy
4	Marked	Posterior pole details barely visible
5	Severe	Posterior pole not visible

yellow-white, raised, or flat lesions with blurred margins. Lesions may be single or multiple, large or small. Grading of severity is based on the extent of retinal and choroidal involvement rather than on the activity of each lesion. Inactive, healed lesions are not scored.

Neovascularization

Neovascularization may be preretinal or subretinal. Only active, new vessel growth is scored as present for each quadrant (NVE). Neovascularization of the disc (NVD) is scored separately (see later discussion). Inactive, regressed vessels or mature vessels in fibroglial outgrowths are not scored.

Lesions of the disc and macula are included within the fundus score, separately from the vitreous and the anterior segment scores. Inflammation of the disc (papillitis) is graded on a scale of 1 to 3, whereas NVD is scored as absent or present. Edema of the macula is also recorded as absent or present on the basis of macular thickening or cystoid changes as seen through slit-lamp biomicroscopy.

Visual Acuity

Visual acuity is probably the most important parameter in determining the efficacy of any new drug therapy. However, visual acuity for distance and near is scored and recorded separately and independent from inflammation scores. It is possible that obvious reduction in macular edema may occur without definite improvement in the degree of intraocular inflammation. Thus, changes in visual acuity need not parallel exactly the changes in the degree of inflammation.

Fluorescein Angiography

In cases of posterior uveitis in which the media are relatively clear and the degree of vitreous haze is not marked, fluorescein angiography of the fundus may be helpful in evaluating the extent of retinal inflammation. As for the clinical observations, no attempt to grade the severity of the individual inflammatory signs from the fluorescein angiographic data should be made. A prototype grading system for the evaluation of inflammatory activity of fluo-

UVEITIS SCORING SHEET

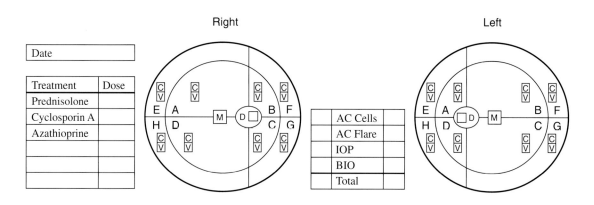

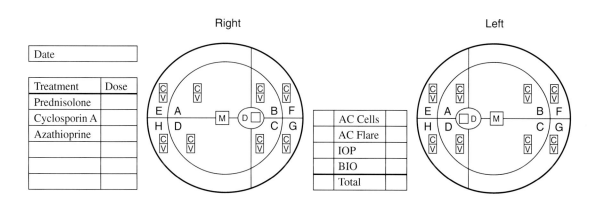

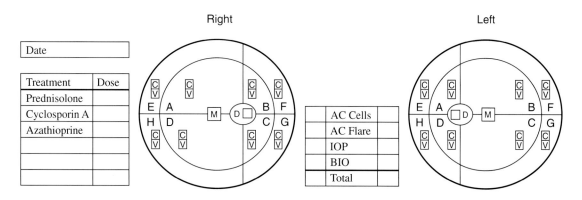

Figure 2.2. Uveitis scoring sheet

Name _____   Date _____

SCORING SHEET # 2 – FLUORESCEIN ANGIOGRAPHY

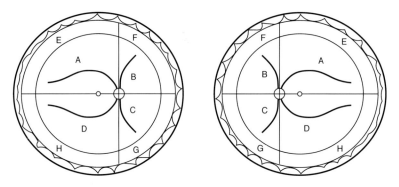

0, 1 = Focal, 2 = Sector, 3 = Diffuse, *0 = No, 1 = Yes

1. Retinal vessel leakage (0–3)   _____

2. Optic disc vessel leakage (0, 1)*   _____

3. Macular edema (0, 1)*   _____

4. Capillary dropout (0–3)   _____

5. Arteriolar occlusion (0–3)   _____

6. Venule occlusion (0–3)   _____

7. Late staining of vessels (0–3)   _____

8. Retinochoroidal infiltrates (0–3)   _____

9. Retinal neovascularization (0–3)   _____

10. Disc neovascularization (0, 1)*   _____

11. Subretinal neovascularization (0–3)   _____

– Focal lesions are unique and < 1DD, while sector are > 1DD and are within one quadrant, and diffuse are in more than one quadrant. The late frames of the angiogram are best to look for increasing hyperfluorescence as evidence of activity.

Figure 2.3. Scoring sheet #2–fluorescein angiography

rescein angiograms is suggested. The fundus is divided into quadrants as previously outlined. It is likely that most angiograms will be directed toward the postequatorial fundus. In cases of peripheral retinal vasculitis, peripheral quadrant views may be taken in the late stages, because these views would be most informative in demonstrating signs of the activity. The number of inflammatory signs that can be separately graded is greater on fluorescein angiography. For certain lesions scoring is based on whether the lesion is absent or present. For other lesions the extent of the lesion is graded in each quadrant according to whether the lesion is focal (< 1 disc diameter in size) or sectorial (> 1 disc diameter in size). Diffuse lesions are those that occur in more than one quadrant (focal or sectorial).

General Approach to Scoring

Each of the components, that is, anterior segment, vitreous, fundus, visual acuity, and fluorescein angiography, should be scored separately, and attempts at summating the scores should not be made. Moreover, a maximum score for any one of the components reflects solely on the relative inflammatory activity of the other components no matter how high the separate score of each component.

The uveitis scoring system described here emphasizes only those features that represent signs of disease activity that can be readily and simply recorded on standard forms in the clinic. The anterior segment is examined using a Haag-Streit slit lamp or equivalent instrument, and the posterior segment is examined with a binocular indirect ophthalmoscope. Examination of the macula may be performed with a +60 to +90 aspheric lens, a Hruby lens, or a contact lens under the slit lamp. The presence of an active lesion in any quadrant of the fundus is noted in a diagram. Codes are written in each quadrant of the diagram for each type of lesion (v = vasculitis; c = choroidoretinal infiltrate; n = neovascularization). Further information can be added by drawing the findings on the diagram. This, however, is only descriptive and does not add to the overall score.

Epilogue

After a few years of open and masked studies evaluating the effectiveness of drug therapy in endogenous uveitis, it was realized that adequate and reproducible evaluation of the intraocular inflammatory activity was not possible with the current system. Therefore, based on the accumulated experience of the authors, a scoring system of grading is suggested. We believe that this system may be useful in assessing the effectiveness of drug therapy. Moreover, it is possible that this scoring system may be used to identify the clinical effects of drugs. Thus, a better assessment of a therapy regimen as well as a more specific treatment may be achieved.

It is our hope that widespread use of this scoring system would enhance both understanding of the basic pathologic process in uveitis and the efficacy of therapeutic regimens. Last but not least, we believe that the use of this scoring system is essential for studies aimed at assessing the beneficial therapeutic potential of any new drug for the treatment of endogenous uveitis.

Uveitis Scoring System

Anterior Segment

	SCORE
Ciliary injection	Absent = 0
	Present = 1
Anterior chamber	
Cells	0 = nil: < 5 cells
	1 = mild: 5–10 cells
	2 = moderate: 11–20 cells
	3 = marked: 21–50 cells
	4 = severe: > 50 cells
	5 = severe: hypopyon
Flare	0 = nil to trace
	1 = mild: clearly noticeable, visible
	2 = moderate: without plastic aqueous
	3 = marked: with plastic aqueous
	4 = severe: heavy with fibrin deposits or clots (iris details hazy)

Vitreous

BIO: HAZE = CELLS AND EXUDATE

0 = nil

1 = minimal: posterior pole clearly visible

2 = mild: posterior pole details slightly hazy

3 = moderate: posterior pole shows very hazy details

4 = marked: details of posterior pole are obscured

5 = severe: no details are visible

Fundus

1. Retinal vasculitis
   Regions: A–H
   Activity: Absent = 0
              Present = 1
2. Chorioretinal lesions
   Regions: A–H
   Activity: Absent = 0
              Present = 1

   Macular edema
      Absent = 0
      Present = 1
   Optic Papillitis
      0 = nil
      1 = mild: hyperemia
      2 = moderate: hyperemia and hemorrhages
      3 = severe: elevation of disc, infiltration

Summary of Scoring

COMPONENT	MAXIMUM SCORE	
Anterior segment		
Ciliary injection	1	
Anterior chamber		
Cells	5	
Flare	4	
		Total = 10
Vitreous		
Haze	5	
		Total = 5
Fundus		
Retinal vasculitis	8	
Chorioretinal lesions	8	
		Total = 16
Macula		
Edema	1	
		Total = 1
Papillitis	3	
		Total = 3
Retinal neovascularization		
NVD (0 or 1)	1	
NVE (0 or 1)		
quadrants A, B,		
C, D, E, F, G, H	8	
		Total = 9

Comments

Anterior Segment

1. Anterior chamber cells are determined using the narrowest slit beam (0.5 mm) at 8 mm high at maximum luminance. Pigment and red blood cells are to be ignored.
2. Anterior chamber flare is determined using the narrowest slit beam 0.5 mm at highest luminance. Refer to standard photographs/illustrations (see Figure 2.1).
3. Secondary features such as keratic precipitates, synechiae, iris vessel dilatation and rubeosis, iris nodules, and secondary corneal changes can be noted but do not add to the score.

Vitreous

Vitreous haze is determined by binocular indirect ophthalmoscopy using a 20-diopter lens to observe the posterior pole. Vitreal activity can range from the greatest amount of activity (5+), to the lesser intermediate points of 4+, to trace, to no evidence of vitreal haze at all (0). A 3+ vitreal haze is one in which the optic nerve head is obscured. A 2+ vitreal haze would permit the observer to see the optic nerve head but the borders are not distinct. A 1+ haze permits better visualization of the retinal vessels, and a 0 haze permits a better definition of both the optic nerve head and the retinal vessels. The difference between 1+ vitreal haze and 0 would be that in trace eyes there is slight blurring of the optic disc margin because of the haze, and the normal striations and reflex of the nerve fiber layer cannot be visualized. This assessment may be limited by the presence of lenticular or corneal opacities, hypotony, and recurrent vitreal hemorrhage.[10]

Fundus

1. Although it is expected that many departments will automatically undertake fluorescein angiography where possible, this modality has been excluded from the current scoring system. Fluorescein angiography is mandatory in fully evaluating the extent of retinal disorders and subretinal neovascularization and should be

used where possible. A scoring system integrating this modality is being prepared.

2. Retinal vasculitis is graded as present or absent in the various quadrants, based on activity. Indications of activity would include the following:

    Venous engorgement
    Caliber change
    Hemorrhages but not vascular occlusion
    Vascular occlusion
    Venous or arterial ± cotton wool spots
    Arterial and venous occlusion
    Severe retinal edema
    Necrosis

3. Macular edema is marked as either present or absent. It is preferable to use either a +90D, +60D, Hruby, or contact lens.

4. Neovascularization is a sequel to the inflammatory disease but in itself can represent a dynamic feature of the disease because it can change in response to therapy or simply in the course of the disease. Accordingly, neovascularization on the disc (NVD) is scored arbitrarily as 0 for absent and 1 for present, whereas neovascularization elsewhere (NVE) in any of the quadrants (A–H) is scored 0 for absent and 1 for present. Subretinal neovascularization should be assessed by fluorescein angiography.   .

General Approach to Scoring

Each of the above features needs to be scored separately, and attempts at summating the scores should not be made. This is because patients with severe disease such as Grade 5 vitreous haze might have retinal vasculitis, which would not be assessable because of obscuration of fundal details. Therefore, any quantitative assessment should look at each aspect separately, that is, anterior segment disease, vitreous disease, fundal disease, macular disease, optic nerve disease, and neovascularization. Visual acuity also should be scored separately. A situation therefore might be envisaged in which a patient's anterior chamber and vitreous inflammation respond to therapy but their retinal vasculitis or neovascularization might remain unchanged. In fact, this will be extremely useful in determining the precise effects of any drug on specific aspects of ocular inflammatory disease. Although fluorescein angiography is not an integral part of this scoring system, it is recommended that a fluorescein angiography be performed.

References

1. BenEzra D: Diseases of the choroid and anterior uvea, in Mechaelson's textbook of the fundus of the eye, 3rd ed. Edinburgh: Churchill Livingston, 1980:667–712.
2. Tabbara K: Chlorambucil in Behcet's diseases: A reappraisal. Ophthalmology 1983;90:906.
3. BenEzra D, Cohen E: Treatment and visual prognosis in Behcet's disease. Br J Ophthalmol 1986;70:589.
4. Nussenblatt RB, Palestine AG, Rook AH, et al.: Treatment of intraocular inflammatory disease with cyclosporin A. Lancet 1983;II:235–238.
5. BenEzra D: Cyclosporin A in Behcet's disease: An overview, in Lehner, T, Barnes CS (eds): Recent advances in Behcet's disease. London: Royal Society of Medicine Services, London, 1986:319–325.
6. Towler HMA, Cliffe AM, Whiting PH, Forrester JV: Low dose cyclosporin A therapy in chronic posterior uveitis. Eye 1989;3:282–287.
7. BenEzra D, Cohen E, Chajek T, et al.: Evaluation of conventional therapy versus cyclosporin A in Behcet's syndrome. Transplant Proc 1988;20:136.
8. Hogan MD, Kimura SJ, Thygeson P: Signs and symptoms of uveitis. I. Anterior uveitis. Am J Ophthalmol 1989;47:155.
9. Kimura SJ, Thygeson P, Hogan MD: Signs and symptoms of uveitis. I. Classifications of the posterior manifestations of uveitis. Am J Ophthalmol 1959;47:177.
10. Nussenblatt RB, Palestine AG, Chan CC, Roberge F: Standardization of vitreal inflammatory activity in intermediate and posterior uveitis. Ophthalmology 1985;92:467–471.
11. Forrester JV: Chronic intraocular inflammation. Trans Ophthalmol Soc UK 1985;104:250–255.
12. Forrester JV, Liversidge J, Dua HS, et al.: Comparison of clinical and experimental uveitis. Cur Eye Res 1990;9 suppl:75–84.
13. Kiljstra K, Luydenijk L, van der Gaag R, et al.: IgG and IgA immune response against klebsiella in HLA-B27 associated anterior uveitis. Br J Ophthalmol 1986;70:85–88.
14. BenEzra D: Bilateral anterior uveitis and interstitial nephritis. Am J Ophthalmol 1988;106:766.
15. Chan C-C, BenEzra D, Rodriguez MM, et al.: Immunohistochemistry and electron microscopy of choroidal infiltrates and Dalen-Fuchs nodules in sympathetic ophthalmia. Ophthalmology 1985;92:580.
16. Chan C-C, BenEzra D, Hsu SM, et al.: Immunohistochemical characterization of the granulomas in sympathetic ophthalmia and sarcoidosis. Arch Ophthalmol 1985;103:198.

17. Inomata H, Sakamoto T: Immunopathological studies of Vogt-Koyanagi-Harada disease with sunset sky fundus. Curr Eye Res 1990;9 suppl:35–40.
18. Sharp DC, Bell RA, Patterson E, Pikerton RMH: Sympathetic ophthalmia: Histopathologic and fluorescein angiographic correlation. Arch Ophthalmol 1984;102: 232–235.
19. BenEzra D: Inflammations of the retina and its vessels, in Michaelson's textbook of the fundus of the eye, 3rd ed. Edinburgh: Churchill-Livingston, 1980:3 51–388.
20. Metamoros N, BenEzra D: Bilateral retinopathy and encephalopathy. Graefe's Arch Clin Exp Ophthalmol 1989;227:39.
21. Jakobiec F, Marboe C, Knowles D, et al.: Human sympathetic ophthalmia. Ophthalmology 1983;90: 76–71.
22. Chan C-C, Mochizuki M, Palestine AG, et al.: Kinetics of T-lymphocyte subsets in the eyes of Lewis rats with experimental autoimmune uveitis. Cell Immunol 1985; 96:430.
23. Inomata H: Necrotic changes of choroidal melanocytes in sympathetic ophthalmia. Arch Ophthalmol 1988; 106:239–242.

II
Infectious Diseases

Chapter 3
Viral Infections

Khalid F. Tabbara

A number of viruses can affect the posterior segment of the eye and lead to posterior uveitis. Viruses may lead to damage of the retina, choroid, or optic nerve either by direct invasion or as a result of immunologically mediated mechanisms.[1,2]

Human Immune Deficiency Virus

Acquired immune deficiency syndrome (AIDS) is a disease caused by human immune deficiency virus (HIV). The incidence of AIDS has been increasing over the past decade throughout the world. Homosexuals and drug addicts are more commonly affected by HIV infection than are other individuals. More than 250,000 cases of AIDS and 150,000 deaths of AIDS have been reported in the United States. The World Health Organization estimates that the number of patients infected with HIV will be 20 million in the year 2000.

Transmission of Human Immunodeficiency Virus

The human immunodeficiency virus is transmitted by sexual contact (homosexual and heterosexual), sharing of intravenous needles, perinatal transmission, occupational transmission, and blood and blood product transmissions. The risk of an HIV-positive mother transmitting infection to her infant at or before birth is 25% to 40%. Breast feeding has also resulted in transmission of HIV to infants. Estimates for the risk of HIV infection after a simple needle prick exposure by health personnel is 0.4%.

Clinical Findings

The eye is a commonly involved organ in patients suffering from AIDS.[3] There are two aspects of the ocular manifestations of AIDS: (1) The clinical manifestations caused by the HIV infection of the ocular structures and (2) the clinical findings secondary to the invasion of the ocular structures by opportunistic organisms. The role of the ophthalmologist is twofold: first, to assist the internist in making the diagnosis of the systemic infection, and second, to manage vision-threatening lesions resulting from opportunistic infection that may lead to blindness.

HIV Infection of the Eye. The eye appears to be a unique target of injury by many infectious agents in patients with AIDS, starting with the ocular surface structures. HIV has been isolated from tears of patients with AIDS. This has created some concern among ophthalmologists because of the use of contact lens fitting sets. Hydrogen peroxide appears to be adequate for sterilization of the contact lens. In the normal population, Kaposi's sarcoma of the conjunctiva is rare, but in patients with AIDS, Kaposi's sarcoma is common. Among 201 patients with this disorder who were seen at the San Francisco General Hospital from 1983 to 1986, all patients were homosexual males except for three who were intravenous drug abusers (one female and two male patients).[4] The age range of this group of patients was 20 to 68 years. Eye findings occur in two-thirds of patients with AIDS. Kaposi's sarcoma of the conjunctiva or lids may be seen in 20% of the patients. Kaposi's sarcoma of the skin of the eyelid has a typical violaceous discoloration. Histologically it shows the typical spindle cells with sinusoidal cavities of capillary endothelial cell origin. Microangiopathy of the retinal blood vessels is common in patients with AIDS.

Human immunodeficiency virus affects capillaries of the retinal nerve fiber layer, resulting in focal ischemia and swelling of the nerve fiber layer leading to cotton-wool spots (Figure 3.1). Retinal hemorrhages may occur, giving rise to a picture similar to that seen in systemic lupus erythematosus or hypertension. This form of microvasculopathy may be transient in patients with HIV infection.[2,3]

Ocular Changes Caused by Opportunistic Organisms. There are four groups of opportunistic organisms that may afflict the eye. These are (1) parasites; (2) fungi; (3) bacteria; and (4) viruses.

PARASITES.   The most frequently encountered parasite that can afflict the posterior segment of the eye in patients with AIDS is toxoplasmosis. The diagnosis is typically made on the basis of morphology of the lesion. There are two types of ocular toxoplasmosis: (1) The recurrence of an old toxoplasmic disease, in which toxoplasma cysts that in-fect the retinal cells rupture, releasing toxoplasmas, and (2) acquired systemic toxoplasmosis with parasitemia leading to multiple foci of necrotizing retinitis. Ocular toxoplasmosis in patients with AIDS produces severe extensive retinochoroiditis leading to widespread damage to the retina and choroid.[5]

FUNGI.   The most commonly encountered fungus among patients with AIDS is *Candida albicans.* The disease may be related to exacerbation of latent candida organisms found in the mucosa or caused by *de novo* infection by candida or direct intravenous injection of candida by unsterilized needles shared among drug addicts. After candidemia, the organism reaches the choroid and then the retina, causing focal retinitis. The lesion is typically whitish and elevated. Whitish round exudates in the vitreous over the internal limiting membrane may be seen causing the string-of-pearls sign. The vitreous can be invaded by candida, leading to clouding of the vitreous. Microscopic examination of a vitreous biopsy specimen may show pseudohyphae of candida.

Cryptococcus neoformans may cause retinochoroiditis associated with meningitis. *Pneumocystis carinii* may cause choroiditis in patients with AIDS.[6–8] The organism causes interstitial infiltrates in the lung and may lead to fatal pneumonia.

BACTERIAL INFECTIONS.   Mycobacterial infection of the posterior segment leads to predominant choroiditis; (1) *Mycobacterium avium complex,*

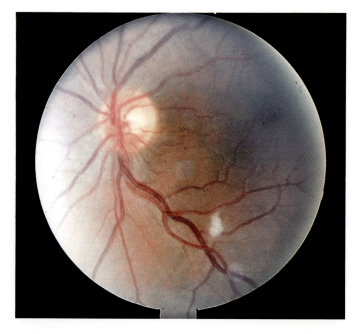

Figure 3.1. Photograph showing a cotton-wool spot in a 23-year-old man with Acquired Immune Deficiency Syndrome.

consisting of the closely related species *M. avium* and *M. intracellulare,* which also can produce patchy choroiditis, and (2) *Mycobacterium tuberculosis.*[9]

Another bacterial infection seen in patients with AIDS is syphilis. Syphilis may cause anterior granulomatous uveitis and roseola of the iris. The posterior segment is involved in the secondary stage of syphilis and consists of retinitis and papillitis.

VIRAL INFECTIONS. Several viruses can produce intraocular lesions in patients with AIDS. Herpes simplex virus (HSV) and varicella-zoster virus (VZV) may affect the posterior segment in patients with AIDS. Acute retinal necrosis is caused by either HSV or VZV. Herpes simplex can affect the retina, causing diffuse arteritis and focal areas of necrosis.[10] Cytomegalovirus (CMV) is a common cause of viral infection of the retina in patients with AIDS.[2-4] CMV retinitis is seen in 15% to 30% of patients with AIDS and is associated with retinal hemorrhages and retinal vasculitis. The CMV retinitis may be associated with retinal hemorrhages. It appears that HIV causes a localized activation of the CMV retinitis, but it is not well understood why patients with AIDS have a tendency to develop CMV infections. Treatment of CMV retinitis is with intravenous (IV) ganciclovir or foscarnet. The retinitis responds to treatment, but patients may have to be placed on maintenance therapy. When treatment is discontinued, lesions may show exacerbation. Intravitreal injections of ganciclovir have been recommended for patients suffering from CMV retinitis.[11]

Laboratory Diagnosis

Patients with AIDS develop positive serology for HIV antibodies and also show a decrease in the T-helper lymphocyte subsets.

Treatment of HIV-Infected Patients

Several drugs have been used in the treatment of HIV-infected patients. Patients with levels of CD4 lymphocytes less than 500 cells/μL should begin on anti-HIV chemotherapy. Rapid loss of CD4 lymphocytes (> 100 cells/μL/year) is another indication for the initiation of anti-HIV therapy. Treatment consists of Zidovudine (AZT, Retrovir, Burroughs Wellcome Co., Research Triangle Park, NC) 200

Table 3.1. Differentiation between Acute Retinal Necrosis (ARN) and Progressive Outer Retinal Necrosis (PORN)

	ARN	PORN
Symptoms	Pain and decrease in vision	Decrease in vision
Location	Peripheral	Peripheral + macular
Course	Rapid	Rapid
Anterior uveitis	Present	Absent
Vasculitis	Occlusive vasculitis	No vasculitis
Recurrence	No recurrence	Recurrence

mg orally six times daily or 500 mg orally three times daily. Postexposure prophylaxis consists of 200 mg orally every 4 hours for 3 days then 200 mg orally five times daily for 4 weeks. The FDA has approved the use of AZT in pregnant women to prevent the disease in the fetus.

Another anti-HIV drug is didanosine (ddI, Videx), which is given to patients who show deterioration on AZT. The drug can be used in combination or alternately with AZT. ddI is given 300 mg orally twice daily for patients over 75 kg. Patients who weigh 50 to 74 kg may be given ddI 200 mg orally twice a daily. Patients weighing 35 to 49 kg are given ddI 125 mg orally twice daily.

Zalcitibine (ddC, Hivid) can be given in combination with AZT at a dosage level of 0.375 to 0.75 mg orally three times daily. Stavudine (d4T) is an investigational anti-HIV drug from Bristol-Meyers-Squibb (Evansville, IN). Stavudine (d4T) was recently approved by the Food and Drug Administration for use in patients with AIDS who show evidence of deterioration on AZT.

Subacute Sclerosing Panencephalitis

Subacute sclerosing panencephalitis (SSPE) is a disease associated with chronic measles virus infection. The virus involves the central nervous system.

Clinical Findings

The main systemic clinical findings include the development of stupor, personality changes, and mental deterioration. The neurologic symptoms may precede the onset of retinitis. The predominant ocular findings consist of focal areas of retinitis involving the paramacular area and the retinal periphery. Mild phlebitis may occur. Patients with SSPE also may develop optic atrophy.

Laboratory Diagnosis

Antibodies to measles are elevated in the serum and the cerebrospinal fluid.

Treatment

No treatment is available. Measles vaccination may prevent this disease.

Cytomegalovirus Infection

Cytomegalovirus (CMV) subclinical systemic infection is common. CMV infection leads to chronic retinitis.[11-18] Immunosuppressed patients are susceptible to the development of CMV infection. The disease may be congenital or acquired. The ocular disease in an immunocompromised individual may represent a reactivation of the virus that has been dormant in tissues for many years or it can be attributable to newly acquired CMV infection. Patients on immunosuppressive therapy, or patients with lymphoproliferative malignancies with AIDS, are susceptible to the development of CMV. The increase in the AIDS population has led to a corresponding increase in the incidence of CMV retinitis. It is estimated that 15% to 30% of patients with AIDS develop CMV retinitis, and 7% of AIDS patients present with CMV retinitis.

Clinical Findings

Patients with CMV infection may complain of blurring of vision or seeing floaters. They also may develop scotomatous areas that are usually not associated with pain.

Nongranulomatous anterior uveitis, which is mild in nature, may develop without posterior synechiae.[19] A mild or minimal amount of cells may be seen in the vitreous. An excessive retinitis may occur in the absence of vitritis.[11-13] The major insult occurs in the posterior segment of the eye. Patients with CMV infection may develop a slowly progressive retinitis. The retinal lesions start as localized retinal infiltrates. The lesions may present in one of three major clinical forms: (1) the hemorrhagic form, which is characterized by the presence of yellow, creamy-white retinitis associated with retinal hemorrhages (Figure 3.2), (2) nonhemorrhagic retinitis, which occurs as a slowly progressive yellow-white infiltration of the retina with advancing borders in a brushfire fashion (Figure 3.3), (3) the granular form is characterized by dry infiltration of the retina with minimal hemorrhages and vasculitis. Involvement of the optic nerve head may occur in both forms of the disease.[11-13] Central vision is lost when the macula is involved. Retinal phlebitis and perivascular sheathing are frequently observed in patients with CMV retinitis. New foci of CMV retinitis are seen in patients with AIDS.

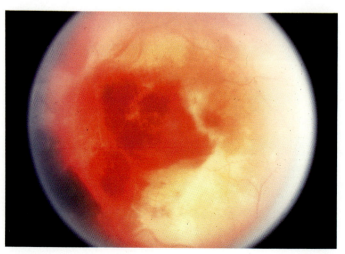

Figure 3.2. Photograph showing cytomegalovirus retinitis (hemorrhagic form). Note the creamy-white infiltration of the retina and the retinal hemorrhages.

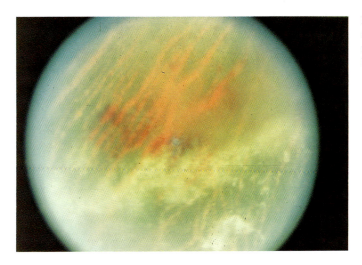

Figure 3.3. Photograph showing cytomegalovirus retinitis (nonhemorrhagic form). Note the brushfirelike advancing borders and lack of vitritis.

The retinitis may lead to focal necrosis (Figure 3.4) in the retina with the development of retinal holes associated with relentless progression. Patients may later develop rhegmatogenous retinal detachment with large necrotic retinal tears that occur in approximately one-fifth of the patients with CMV retinitis. Congenital CMV infection may lead to diffuse or geographic retinitis.

Laboratory Diagnosis

Cytomegalovirus antibody testing is not helpful because CMV infection is common in the general population and false-negative tests in the presence of CMV retinitis may occur. Immunosuppressed individuals may show a decrease in the CD4 cells with helper-to-suppressor's ratio of less than 1. Virus may be cultured from a buffy coat of the blood or from the vitreous when placed on fibroblast cell lines. The diagnosis of CMV retinitis is clinical.

Treatment

Cytomegalovirus may be treated with ganciclovir, which is a virostatic analog of acyclovir. Acyclovir is not effective against the thymidine kinase–negative CMV. Ganciclovir suppresses CMV replication and must be given intravenously every 12 hours.[14–16,20–22] The induction regimen is 5 mg/kg given IV every 12 hours for 14 to 21 days. The maintenance regimen consists of 5 mg/kg daily dose given IV indefinitely. In AIDS patients recur-

rences are common. The main side effects of ganciclovir are bone marrow suppression, neutropenia, and azospermia. Intravitreal injection of ganciclovir may be given at a dosage level of 100 to 200 µg given in 0.1 mL buffered saline solution (BSS) twice weekly initially and then once a week during the maintenance phase.[10,23]

Other therapeutic modalities for CMV infections of the retina include foscarnet, which is given at an initial dose of 60 mg/kg/day three times daily for 3 weeks and a maintenance dose of 100 mg/kg/day IV. Foscarnet is nephrotoxic. Laser treatment is unsuccessful in CMV retinitis.[24–26]

Herpes Simplex and Varicella-Zoster Virus–Necrotizing Retinopathy

Herpes simplex and varicella-zoster virus (VZV) infection may lead to blinding involvement of the posterior segment of the eye. Both acute retinal necrosis syndrome (ARN) and progressive outer segment necrosis (PORN) syndrome may lead to necrotizing retinitis in immunologically competent patients (Figures 3.5–3.8) The disease is caused by hematogenous spread and replication of the virus in the retinal cells. ARN is more common in patients with AIDS than the general population, and PORN has been described in AIDS patients only (see Table 3.1).

Acute Retinal Necrosis Syndrome

Patients with acute ARN caused by herpes simplex either types I or II or VZV complain of a

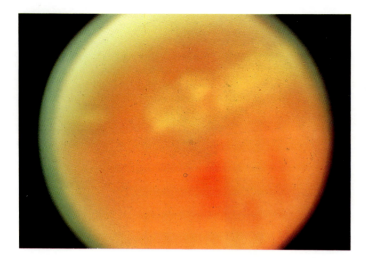

Figure 3.4. A, Photograph showing cytomegalovirus retinitis. **B,** Photograph showing a typical large cytomegalovirus-infected cell with eosinophilic cytoplasmic inclusion in the vitreous of a patient with cytomegalovirus infection.

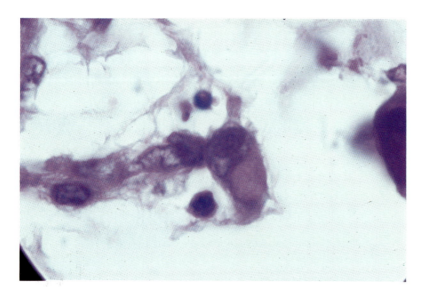

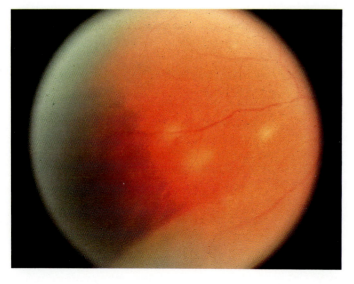

Figure 3.5. Photograph showing acute retinal necrosis. Note the multifocal retinitis.

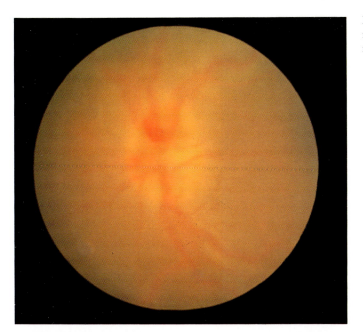

Figure 3.6. Photograph showing acute retinal necrosis. Shows hyperemia of the optic nerve head and vitreous exudates.

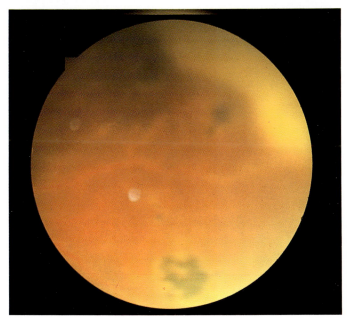

Figure 3.7. Photograph showing acute retinal necrosis. Note the transition zone between normal and the involved necrotized peripheral retina and occlusive vasculitis.

sudden loss of vision associated with redness, pain, and photophobia. Patients also may complain of periorbital pain and pain on moving the globe. Patients may develop floaters and blurring of vision.

Acute retinal necrosis is characterized by focal well-demarcated areas of retinal necrosis in the peripheral retina with evidence of vitreous exudates and cells. The eye shows yellow-white peripheral necrotizing retinitis with relative sparing of the posterior segment of the eye. Occlusive vasculitis is common. The optic nerve head appears to be edematous, and there is evidence of diffuse retinal arteritis. Spontaneous resolution of the retinitis occurs within 5 to 6 weeks. Patients may develop rhegmatogenous retinal detachments, which occurs in 75% of eyes. Patients may lose vision despite aggressive antiviral therapy.

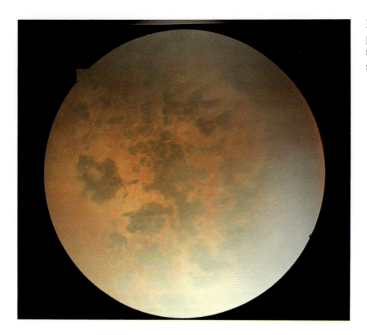

Figure 3.8. Photograph showing same patient as in Figure 3.7, taken 1 year after treatment. Pigmented retinochoroiditic scars are noted.

In rare cases the herpes simplex and VZV retinal necrosis may be associated with evidence of dermatitis. VZV may cause choroiditis.[27] Kelly and Rosenthal[27] reported a 27-year-old woman who developed chorioretinitis secondary to chickenpox (see Table 3.2).

Progressive Outer Retinal Necrosis Syndrome

Progressive outer retinal necrosis syndrome (PORN) is another necrotizing retinopathy that affects patients with AIDS. PORN is the second most common infection of the retina after CMV.

Forster and co-workers[28] described two patients at the University of Southern California who developed rapidly progressive outer retinal necrosis caused by VZV. The two patients developed characteristic involvement of the outer retina with sparing of the retinal vasculature and inner retina until late in the course of the disease. Patients showed poor response to acyclovir given intravenously and developed rhegmatogenous retinal detachment. Retinal biopsy specimen of one patient was examined by electron microscopy and showed hexagonally shaped virus particles measuring 100 nm in diameter consistent with herpes virus. Polymerase chain reaction demonstrated herpes virus in the retinal biopsy specimen of the second patient.[28] Margolis and associates,[29] described the histopathologic

Table 3.2. Differentiation between Varicella-Zoster Virus (VZV) and Cytomegalovirus (CMV) Retinitis

	VZV	**CMV**
Course	Rapid	Slow
Visual loss	Severe visual loss	Variable
Lesions	Multifocal	1–3 lesions/eye
Retinal detachment	Detachment majority	Retinal detachment in 20%
CD4	0–100	0–50
	Deep retinal lesion	Dry granular border
	Clearing around blood vessels	Vasculitis and perivascular sheating
Vasculitis	No vascular occlusion	Vascular occlusion
Treatment	Foscarnet (or high dose acyclovir)	Foscarnet (or ganciclovir)

studies of retinal sections in patients with PORN and demonstrated herpes zoster particles by *in situ* hybridization. Atypical clinical features of ARN and PORN have been described in patients with AIDS.

The two disorders acute retinal necrosis and progressive outer retinal necrosis may represent clinical variants of varicella-zoster retinopathy. The variation in the clinical manifestations of patients with necrotizing herpetic retinopathy does not indicate different clinical entities. The ocular manifestations are related to the strain and type of virus, the immunologic status of the host, and genetic factors.[31–33] These factors play a role in the pathogenesis of the disease and its clinical manifestations.

Patients with PORN present with painless rapid deterioration of vision. Patients may complain of dimming of vision, and the visual acuity may decrease with time. Peripheral foci of retinitis are noted with little inflammation and deep retinal opacification. The condition may involve the central macular.

Patients develop rapidly progressive homogenous creamy lesions of the retina with outer retinal necrosis. PORN shows thick opaque scarring with cracks that can be differentiated from fine pigment stipplings in the fundus of patients with CMV retinitis.

The clinical picture of PORN consists of multifocal retinitis with cherry-red spots. The lesions show a tendency to coalesce. No occlusive vasculitis or perivascular sheathing are seen. Perivascular lucid areas with retinal detachment may occur. Thick plaques are sometimes noted. PORN is therefore characterized by peripheral and posterior rapid necrosis with little inflammation and no anterior uveitis.

The Education and Research Committee of the American Uveitis Society has developed criteria for diagnosis of the necrotizing herpetic retinopathy disorders and recommended that the term "necrotizing herpetic retinopathy" be used for retinal lesions presumed to be caused by one of the herpes viruses.[30] The criteria are outlined as follows:

American Uveitis Society Criteria for
Diagnosis of the Acute Retinal Necrosis
Syndrome and Other Necrotizing
Herpetic Retinopathies[*30]

The Education and Research Committee of the American Uveitis Society has developed the following terminology and definitions for use in research and publications dealing with necrotizing viral retinopathies that are presumed or proven to be caused by one of the herpesviruses.

   A. The umbrella designation, "necrotizing herpetic retinopathy," should be used for retinal lesions presumed to be caused by one of the herpesviruses (herpes simplex virus, varicella-zoster virus, or cytomegalovirus), when the specific causal agent is not known and the characteristics of the lesion do not fit all criteria for a well-defined clinical syndrome, such as cytomegalovirus retinitis or acute retinal necrosis syndrome (see B below). The term, necrotizing herpetic retinopathy, should replace terms such as atypical acute retinal necrosis or limited acute retinal necrosis.

B. Criteria for use of the term, acute retinal necrosis syndrome, are as follows:

   1. A designation of acute retinal necrosis syndrome should be based solely on clinical appearance and course of infection. Clinical characteristics that must be seen include:

      a. One or more focus of retinal necrosis with discrete borders located in the peripheral retina (primarily involving the area adjacent to, or outside of, the major temporal vascular arcades). Macular lesions, although less common, do not preclude a diagnosis of acute retinal necrosis syndrome if they occur in the presence of peripheral lesions.

      b. Rapid progression of disease (advancement of lesion borders or development of new foci of necrosis) if antiviral therapy has not been given.

      c. Circumferential spread of disease.

      d. Evidence of occlusive vasculopathy with arteriolar involvement.

      e. A prominent inflammatory reaction in the vitreous and anterior chamber.

   2. Characteristics that support, but are not required for, a diagnosis of acute retinal necrosis syndrome include:

      a. Optic neuropathy/atrophy.

      b. Scleritis.

      c. Pain.

   3. The definition of acute retinal necrosis syndrome does not depend on the extent of necrosis. As long as the criteria in B1 (a–e) are met, the disease can be designated acute retinal necrosis syndrome, and modifiers such as "limited" are not necessary.

Source: Holland GN: Standard diagnostic criteria for the acute retinal necrosis syndrome. *Am J Ophthalmol* 1994;117:663–667.

4. The definition of acute retinal necrosis syndrome does not depend on the gender, age, race, or immunologic status of the host.

5. Because it is based on the clinical appearance and course of disease only, the designation of acute retinal necrosis syndrome is not influenced by isolation of any virus or other pathogen from ocular tissues of fluid. If lesions do not meet the criteria outlined in B1 (a–e), the disease should not be referred to as acute retinal necrosis syndrome whether or not varicella-zoster virus is isolated from the eye.

C. If a causal agent is identified (for example, by microscopic examination of biopsy specimens, vitreous culture, evidence of intraocular antibody production, or polymerase chain reaction techniques), then the retinopathy should be referred to as being caused by the agent. If it also fits the diagnostic criteria for a clinical syndrome, that designation can be included as a modifier, if appropriate for the situation in which it is being discussed. Serum antibody titers are not a reliable means of making a causal diagnosis. Because of its highly characteristic appearance, cytomegalovirus retinitis in patients with AIDS or other immunodeficiency states would remain a clinically defined syndrome yet retain its specific causal designation, even without identification of the virus. In contrast, acute retinal necrosis syndrome and varicella-zoster virus retinitis are not interchangeable terms.

D. Other distinct syndromes may emerge that can be defined clinically. One should not refer to these other clinical syndromes as variants of acute retinal necrosis syndrome; rather they are clinical variants in a spectrum of necrotizing herpetic retinopathy.

Laboratory Diagnosis

Detectable antibody titers for either herpes simplex or VZV may be found. Presence of gamma G immunoglobulin (IgG) antibody for these viruses is common among the general population and, therefore, has limited diagnostic value. Lumbar puncture may show cerebrospinal fluid (CSF) lymphocytosis, and the virus may occasionally be cultured

from the vitreous during the acute phase of the disease or through an eye wall biopsy of the retina and choroid.

Treatment

Treatment of acute retinitis caused by *Herpes simplex* virus or VZV consists of acyclovir 10 mg/kg IV every 8 hours for 10 to 14 days. Intravitreal injection of acyclovir may be given at a dosage level of 75 μg once a week for two to three doses. Patients are later shifted to oral acyclovir 800 mg orally every 6 hours. In case of acyclovir resistance, Foscarnet may be given 40 mg/kg IV by infusion pump every 8 hours for 3 weeks. Repair of the detachment is done through a pars plana lensectomy, vitrectomy, endolaser photocoagulation, and gas tamponade.

Herpetic chorioretinitis may occur in the newborn after infection is acquired by the infant at the time of passage down through the birth canal. Mothers who have herpetic cervicitis at the time of childbirth may be given oral acyclovir therapy. The newborn infant may develop both chorioretinitis and encephalitis as a result of viremia caused by herpes simplex type 2.

Epstein–Barr Virus

Multifocal choroiditis has been seen in patients with systemic Epstein–Barr virus (EBV) infection. No retinal or choroidal biopsy specimens have been obtained. The diagnosis is clinical. The association is circumstantial, and the clinical entity remains to be documented as caused by EBV.

Rubella Chorioretinitis

Rubella chorioretinitis is predominantly a congenital rubella infection that has some similarities to the posterior segment features seen in herpetic chorioretinitis of the newborn.

Clinical Findings

The clinical findings during the active phase of the disease includes focal patches of retinitis in the posterior pole. This is followed by evidence of focal atrophy of the retina and areas of hyperpigmentation. The inflammation may stay active at the time of birth, but it is generally quiescent by the time it is first detected in the fundus of the affected infant. Other ocular findings attributable to rubella include congenital glaucoma, cataract, and microphthalmos. The most severe damage is sustained to the eye when rubella infection is transmitted to the fetus during the first trimester of pregnancy. Other signs of systemic illness caused by rubella may include congenital heart disease, congenital deafness, and neurologic manifestations.

Laboratory Diagnosis

Rubella is a disease that is diagnosed clinically. Neutralizing antibodies can be detected in the mother's blood within 10 days after the infection. A solid-phase radioimmunoassay is also useful for screening. Rubella-specific IgG and IgM antibodies should be determined in the mother and the fetus.

Treatment

No treatment is available for rubella. Prevention is by receiving rubella vaccine.

References

1. Pepose JS: Infectious retinitis: Diagnostic modalities. Ophthalmology 1986;93(5):570–573.
2. Nussenblatt RB, Palestine AG: Uveitis fundamentals and clinical practice. Chicago: Year Book Medical Publishers, 1989.
3. Jabs DA, Green WR, Fox R, et al.: Ocular manifestations of acquired immune deficiency syndrome. Ophthalmology 1989;96(7):1092–1099.
4. O'Donnell J: Personal communication, 1989.
5. Parke DW, Font RL: Diffuse toxoplasmic retinochoroiditis in a patient with AIDS. Arch Ophthalmol 1986;104(4):571–575.
6. Dugel PU, Rao NA, Forster DJ, et al.: Pneumocystis carinii choroiditis after long-term aerosolized pentamidine therapy. Am J Ophthalmol 1990;110(2):113–117.
7. Macher AM, Bardenstein DS, Zimmerman LE, et al.: Pneumocystics carinii choroiditis in a male homosexual with AIDS and disseminated pulmonary and extrapulmonary P. Carinii infection. N Engl J Med 1987;316:1092.
8. Rao NA, Zimmerman PL, Boyer D, et al.: A clinical, histopathologic, and electron microscopic study of pneumocystics carinii choroiditis. Am J Ophthalmol 1989;107(3):218–228.
9. Blodi BA, Johnson MW, McLeish WM, et al.: Presumed choroidal tuberculosis in a human immunodeficiency virus infected host. Am J Ophthalmol 1989;108(5):605–607.
10. Luyendijk L, v.d. Horn GJ, Visser OH, et al.: Detection of locally produced antibodies to herpes viruses in the aqueous of patients with acquired immune deficiency syndrome (AIDS) or acute retinal necrosis syndrome (ARN). Curr Eye Res 1990;9 (suppl):7–11.
11. Freeman WR: Intraocular antiviral therapy. Arch Ophthalmol 1989;107(12):1737–1739.
12. Gross JG, Sadun AA, Wiley CA, et al.: Severe visual lose related to isolated peripapillary retinal and optic nerve head Cytomegalovirus infection. Am J Ophthalmol 1989;108(6):691–698.
13. Hennis HL, Scott AA, Apple DJ: Cytomegalovirus retinitis. Surv Ophthalmol 1989;34(3):193–203.
14. Jennens ID, Lucas CR, Sandland AM, et al.: Cytomegalovirus cultures during maintenance DHPG therapy for cytomegalovirus (CMV) retinitis in acquired immunodeficiency syndrome (AIDS). J Med Virol 1990;30(1):42–44.
15. Kaps D, Daus W, Volcker HE: Ganciclovir (DHPG)-treatment of cytomegalovirus retinitis in AIDS. Fortschr Ophthalmol 1989;86(6):600–603.
16. Kaulfersch W, Urban C, Hauer C, et al.: Successful treatment of CMV retinitis with ganciclovir after allogeneic marrow transplantation. Bone Marrow Transplant 1989;4(5):587–589.
17. LeCalve M, Petroni-Placenta M, Bognaud M, et al.: Clinical aspects of cytomegalovirus necrotizing retinitis in AIDS. Bull Soc Ophthalmol Fr 1988;88(11):1345–1348.
18. Levin AV, Zeichner S, Duker JS, et al.: Cytomegalovirus retinitis in an infant with acquired immunodeficiency syndrome. Pediatrics 1989;(4):683–687.
19. Dyszynska-Rosciszewska B, Drobecka-Brydakowa E, Moszczynska-Kowalska A, et al.: Ocular symptoms in cytomegalovirus infection. Klin Oczna 1988;90(11):391–392.
20. Rosecan LR, Laskin OL, Kalman CM, et al.: Antiviral therapy with ganciclovir for cytomegalovirus retinitis and bilateral exudative retinal detachments in an immunocompromised child. Ophthalmology 1986;93(11):1401–1407.
21. Rosecan LR, Stahl-Bayliss CM, Kalman CM, Laskin, OL: Antiviral therapy for cytomegalovirus retinitis in AIDS with dihydroxy propoxymethyl guanine. Am J Ophthalmol 1986;101(4):405–418.
22. Heinemann MH: Long-term intravitreal ganciclovir therapy for cytomegalovirus retinopathy. Arch Ophthalmol 1989;107(12):1767–1772.
23. Fanning MM, Read SE, Benson M, et al.: Foscarnet therapy of cytomegalovirus retinitis in AIDS. J Acquir Immune Defic Syndr 1990;3(5):472–479.

24. Farese RV Jr, Schambelan M, Hollander H, et al.: Nephrogenic diabetes insipidus associated with foscarnet treatment of cytomegalovirus retinitis. Ann Intern Med 1990;112(12):955–956.

25. Palestine AG, Stevens G Jr, Lane HC, et al.: Treatment of cytomegalovirus retinitis with dihydroxy propoxymethyl guanine. Am J Ophthalmol 1986;101(1): 95–101.

26. Bloom SM, Snady-McCoy L: Multifocal choroiditis uveitis occurring after herpes zoster ophthalmicus. Am J Ophthalmol 1989;108(6):733–735.

27. Kelly SP, Rosenthal AR: Chickenpox choroiditis. Br J Ophthalmol 1990;74:698–699.

28. Forster DJ, Dugel PU, Frangeih GT, et al.: Rapidly progressive outer retinal necrosis in the acquired immunodeficiency syndrome. Am J Ophthalmol 1990;110: 341–348.

29. Margolis TP, Lowder CY, Holland GN, et al.: Varicella-zoster virus retinitis in patients with the acquired immunodeficiency syndrome. Am J Ophthalmol 1991; 112:119.

30. Holland GN: Standard diagnostic criteria for the acute retinal necrosis syndrome. Am J Ophthalmol 1994; 117:663–667.

31. Duker JS, Blumenkranz MS: Diagnosis and management of acute retinal necrosis (ARN) syndrome. Surv Ophthalmol 1991;35:327.

32. Culbertson WW, Blumenkranz MS, Pepose JS, et al.: Varicella-zoster virus is a cause of the acute retinal necrosis syndrome. Ophthalmology 1986;93:559.

33. Holland GN, Cornell PJ, Park MS, et al.: An association between acute retinal necrosis syndrome and HLA-DQw7 and phenotype Bw62, DR4. Am J Ophthalmol 1989;108:370.

Chapter 4
Endogenous Bacterial Infections

Khalid F. Tabbara

Spirochetal Diseases

Spirochetes are a large heterogenous group of motile organisms. The family Spirochaetaceae includes three genera of free-living spiral organisms: (1) Treponema, (2) Borrelia, and (3) Leptospira. All three spirochetes may cause chronic human disease and may infect the host for many years. In addition, all three spirochetes may cause uveitis.

Endemic Syphilis (Bejel)

Endemic syphilis, also known as Bejel, is a non-venereal infection caused by a spirochete that is indistinguishable from *Treponema pallidum*. Some refer to this spirochete as *Treponema pallidum endemicum*. The disease is endemic in many parts of the world but occurs chiefly in Africa, the Middle East, and Southeast Asia. In certain communities 10% to 15% of the population may have positive serology[1]. As in venereal syphilis, humans are the only reservoirs of the infection, and the transmission is principally by direct body contact among children and adults. The onset of the disease is usually in childhood and is characterized by primary skin lesion of buccal mucosal lesions. The primary lesion has a self-limited course, and most patients do not report for medical consultation. The disease may be transmitted by direct body contact and by communal drinking vessels. There have been no cases of congenital bejel reported in the literature. The late stages of the disease may lead to characteristic bony changes, but late neurologic and car-diovascular lesions are uncommon. The initial onset of the disease is characterized by infectious mucous patches with scaly lesions and skin rash. Certain patients may develop the late clinical stages of the disease with gummata formation in bone.

The major diagnostic criteria include: (1) positive serology to *Treponema pallidum*, (2) absence of a primary lesion, (3) skin or characteristic bony changes, (4) history of nonvenereal transmission, (5) absence of history of promiscuity, and (6) absence of cardiovascular and neurologic involvement.[2]

Clinical Findings

Ocular findings in patients with bejel include anterior granulomatous uveitis with posterior synechiae and fibrovascular membrane over the lens in the pupillary area (Figure 4.1). Vitreous may show evidence of opacities. The posterior segment of the eye shows chorioretinitis. Healing is followed by evidence of retinal pigment epithelial proliferation (Figure 4.2). Patients may develop optic atrophy in the late stages of the disease. Some patients may develop areas of choroiditis.[2]

The radiologic examination of patients may show cortical thickening and irregularities in the tibia with gummalike lessions. Subperiosteal new bone formation is common, and bowing of the tibia may occur.[1,2]

Laboratory Diagnosis

Tests for antibodies to *Treponema pallidum* are positive. All tests for syphilis may show positivity in pa-

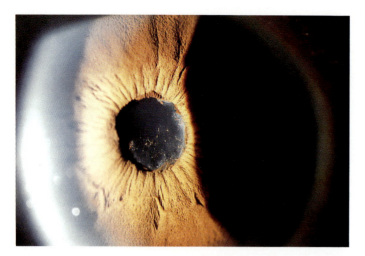

Figure 4.1. Anterior uveitis with posterior syrechiae in a patient with endemic syphilis (Bejel).

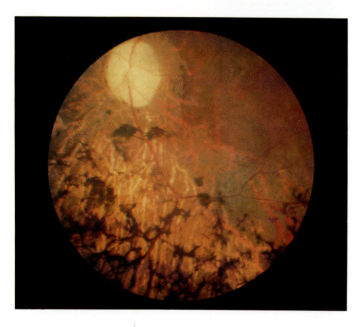

Figure 4.2. Fundus photograph of a 67-year-old patient with healed endemic syphilis showing evidence of optic atrophy and pigmentary changes (pseudoretinitis pigmentosum).

tients with endemic syphilis, including Venereal Disease Research Laboratory (VDRL) test, fluorescent treponemal antibody absorption test (FTA-ABS) and treponemal hemagglutination test (TPHA). Routine serology for nonvenereal syphilis should be performed on patients presenting with uveitis. The endemicity of this condition in certain countries warrants continuous suspicion of the possibility of its occurrence among patients with uveitis. In communities where venereal syphilis may occur, such as the Middle East, India, or Southeast Asia, or East Africa, the differentiation between bejel and syphilis may be extremely difficult to make on serologic

and clinical grounds. Future tests are needed for serologic differentiation between venereal and nonvenereal syphilis. It is postulated, although not confirmed, that endemic syphilis may provide immunity and afford protection to venereal syphilis because of the close antigenicity between *Treponema* causing bejel and *Treponema* causing syphilis. Continuous improvement in socioeconomic status may decrease the problem of Bejel in endemic areas.

Blood for serology by TPHA, VDRL, rapid plasma reagin (RPR), and FTA-ABS are positive in patients with Bejel. Aqueous humor specimens are also found to be positive.[2]

Treatment

Treatment of endemic syphilis consists of the systemic administration of penicillin, tetracycline, or azithromycin. The anterior uveitis also may be treated with topical application of corticosteroid and mydriatics.

The serologic testing for bejel is the same as for syphilis. Furthermore, all tests for syphilis give positive results in patients with Bejel. It is therefore of great clinical importance to be familiar with the entity of endemic syphilis or Bejel. Mistaking Bejel for venereal syphilis can have catastrophic social consequences in conservative societies. Bejel should, in fact, be considered in the differential diagnosis of syphilis.

Syphilis

Syphilis is a disease caused by *Treponema pallidum*. The disease has made great impact on the course of history. Henry VIII, who was infected with syphilis before his marriage, searched for a noninfected wife. When the Catholic Church of Rome refused to sanction his divorce from Catherine of Aragon, Henry VIII countered by renouncing Catholicism and established the church of England, headed by himself. The progeny of Henry VIII, including Mary Tudor (Bloody Mary) and Edward VI, suffered from syphilis and died, opening the door to the reign of Elizabeth and the era of English greatness.

The annual incidence of syphilis throughout the world has declined since the introduction of penicillin. Recently, however, there has been a resurgence of syphilis in Western countries. The incidence has been steadily increasing since the late 1970s among all sexually active populations.[3] In addition, there has been an increase in the incidence of syphilis among homosexual populations and patients with AIDS. There are 40,275 new cases reported every year in the United States alone.

Clinical Findings

Clinical intraocular involvement in syphilis usually occurs during the secondary stage of syphilis. Ocular involvement is less frequent in the tertiary stage of syphilis. The intraocular structures may be involved in the congenital form of the disease. After involvement of the primary site, cutaneous, mucus membrane, or mucocutaneous chancre, the spirochetes disseminate throughout the body, leading to the development of the secondary acquired syphilis (Figures 4.3 and 4.4). Cutaneous manifestations are common in the secondary stage of the disease. Syphilis has been known to mimic any inflammatory disease with ocular involvement.

Acquired Syphilis

Primary syphilis may rarely involve the eyelids, causing a typical chancre. Patients with acquired syphilis may develop anterior or posterior scleritis and sometimes may develop episcleritis. The cornea may be involved in association with the scleral infection. A sclerokeratitis then may occur, and

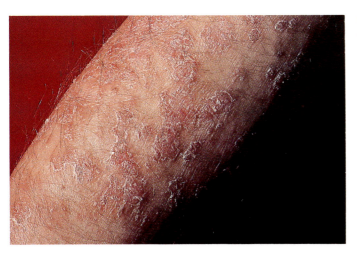

Figure 4.3. A 26-year-old man with secondary syphilis showing papillomacular scaly skin lesions over the arm.

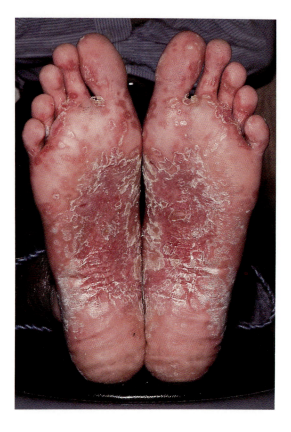

Figure 4.4. Scaly erythematous lesions over the soles in a patient with secondary syphilis.

this may lead to thinning of the sclera. Interstitial keratitis may occur in primary, secondary, and tertiary acquired syphilis and in late congenital syphilis. In acquired syphilis the interstitial keratitis is unilateral, whereas in congenital syphilis the disease is bilateral.

Uveitis is the most ocular manifestation of ocular syphilis.[4,5] Involvement of the uvea and retina occurs in the secondary and tertiary stages of acquired syphilis as well as in the early and late stages of congenital syphilis (Figure 4.5). Patients usually develop an anterior granulomatous or nongranulomatous uveitis. Roseola of the iris may appear in the early stages of secondary syphilis. These are iris papules that are present on the surface of the iris. They may be associated with new vascular tufts that leak fluorescein into the anterior chamber. Synechiae formation is common. Patients develop cutaneous eruptions of the palms or soles that may precede or accompany the anterior uveitis. The iris may become edematous and covered with inflammatory exudates. Fibrin in the anterior chamber, hypopyon, or hemorrhage may be noted. The iris papules may appear yellowish to red in color

and are 0.25 mm in diameter. In congenital syphilis, fibrinous exudates may occur on the surface of the iris, leading to occlusion of the pupil with massive exudation in the vitreous. Severe granulomatous uveitis may lead to phthisis bulbi.

Involvement of the retina and choroid is common in the late secondary stage of syphilis. The involvement may occur also during the gumma formation in the tertiary acquired stage of syphilis. Retinitis and choroiditis also may occur in late congenital syphilis. Involvement consists of focal choroiditis, retinitis, or juxtapapillary chorioretinitis with overlying cellular exudates and vitreous cells.[6] Disseminated syphilitic chorioretinitis is one of the most common ocular manifestation of acquired syphilis. Large areas of placoid chorioretinitis occurs in secondary syphilis. Lesions show early hypofluorescence and late staining by fluorescein angiography. The disease is not responsive to systemic steroid. Chorioretinitis may be unilateral or bilateral. Well-circumscribed areas of inflammation may appear in the posterior segment of the eye, leading to edema of the optic nerve head and retina. Retinal vasculitis is common. Flame-shaped hem-

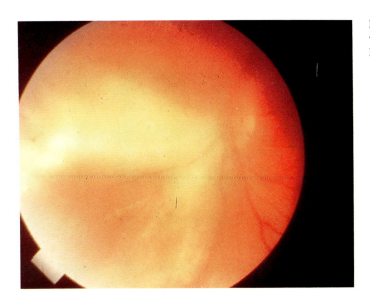

Figure 4.5. Area of retinitis in a patient with secondary syphilis. (Courtesy of Dr. R. Weinberg.)

orrhages may appear with retinitis. Optic neuritis may occur.

The lesions of the posterior segment are characterized by disseminated choroiditis, which may involve the macular area. As the macular lesions heal, the peripheral retina may become involved. Bilateral areolar choroiditis occurs infrequently in late secondary acquired syphilis. The lesions may heal leaving pigmented scars. Atrophic white scars may be seen, which are nummular and surrounded by pigment. Gumma in the choroid and retina are extremely rare. The gumma may occur in the tertiary stage of syphilis and may be associated with focal necrosis.

In patients with congenital syphilis, the disease causes geographic chorioretinitis. Healing leads to areas of pigmentation and depigmentation, and the clinical picture is referred to as the salt and pepper fundus. These lesions are most marked in the periphery of the fundus. Narrowing of the blood vessels and atrophy of the optic nerve may be observed in some patients.

In both acquired and congenital syphilis, optic neuritis may occur. Furthermore, papilledema and involvement of the optic nerve may occur in the late stage of secondary acquired syphilis.

Laboratory Diagnosis

The clinical diagnosis is confirmed by serologic testing. Qualitative and quantitative VDRL and FTA-ABS blood tests should be performed. Other tests for syphilis include RPR and hemagglutination, which are good for screening. Patients with bejel (endemic syphilis)[2] or Lyme disease[7] may show positive serology for syphilis. Patients with HIV infection should be tested for syphilis.[6,8,9]

In the secondary stage of syphilis, cerebrospinal fluid examination should be performed to rule out neurosyphilis. Aqueous humor may be subjected to the determination of antibodies to *Treponema pallidum* and dark field examination for the identification of spirochetes. Certain autoimmune diseases, such as lupus erythematosus, may show false-positive VDRL. The FTA absorption test, however, is specific for syphilis and generally remains positive throughout the lifetime of the patient despite adequate therapy regimen. In the late stages of syphilis, specific antibodies may be found at low titers. Qualitative as well as quantitative titers of antibodies to *Treponema pallidum* should be determined at the time of initial testing. The *Treponema* immobilization test is rarely performed in the general laboratories because of technical difficulties.

Treatment

Treatment of early (primary and secondary) syphilis consists of the administration of benzathine penicillin 2.4 million units intramuscularly (IM) once a week for 3 weeks. If the patient is allergic to penicillin, one may consider the use of doxycycline 100 mg orally twice a day for a period of 4 weeks.

Patients with neurosyphilis should be admitted to the hospital and treated with penicillin-G 12 million units intravenously (IV) daily for 10 days followed by benzathine penicillin 2.4 million units IM once every week for 4 weeks. Probenecid 500 mg orally every 6 hours also may be given to maintain high levels of penicillin. Alternate therapy consists of ceftriaxone 1 g IM daily for 10 days.

Borreliosis (Lyme Disease)

Borreliosis is a systemic disease caused by the Spirochete *Borrelia burgdorferi*. Steere and co-workers identified an epidemic of arthritis among 39 children and 12 adults in Lyme, Connecticut.[10] The illness among the residents of Lyme was characterized by recurring attacks of pain and swelling in the large joints, particularly the knee. Several of the patients of this group had also experienced a characteristic erythematous papule that had developed into a red lesion. This papule was referred to as erythema chronicum migrans, which was first reported in Europe in 1908. After the report of Steere and colleagues, several field studies of both banks of the Connecticut River were carried out.[11] Mammals and deers were collected and examined for ectoparasites. The studies identified a previously unrecorded tick referred to as *Ixodes dammini*, which was reported by Spielman and co-workers from Harvard University.[12] The authors obtained ticks that apparently made a comeback from near extinction. Burgdorfer working at the federal government's Rocky Mountain laboratories in Montana received some of the *Ixodes dammini* sent from Long Island, New York. In 1981, Burgdorfer dissected some of the ticks and examined their midguts and subjected them to dark field microscopy and Giemsa staining. He discovered the presence of a spirochete with structural features similar to those of *Treponema*.[13,14] Burgdorfer studied the spirochetes and established the first animal model of what has become known as the Lyme disease by allowing the *Ixodes dammini* to feed for 12 weeks on rabbits. The rabbits developed macules and papules on their skin. Three to 5 days later the papules enlarged to become elevated annular lesions similar to the erythema chronicum migrans. A few months later, Steere and others found the same spirochete in the blood of Lyme disease victims. In honor of Burgdorfer, the newly discovered Spirochete was named *Borrelia burgdorferi*. Since the initial epidemic in Lyme, Connecticut, several other cases have been reported from the northeastern states as well as from the midwestern and western states. The disease has also been reported from several other countries throughout the world.

Clinical Findings

Lyme disease typically begins with a history of cutaneous eruption consisting of a papule that forms an annular elevation of the skin (erythema chronicum migrans).[15–17] The lesion is accompanied by flulike symptoms consisting of malaise, headache, chills, and fever. This is referred to as the first stage of the disease, which lasts for approximately 4 weeks and is invariably followed by the second stage of musculoskeletal pain, meningeal irritation, cranial nerve and peripheral neuritis, and carditis. In the third stage of the disease, patients experience intermittent monoarticular or oligoarticular inflammation. The arthritis typically involves the large joints, especially the knees.

Ocular Findings

The spirochete *Borrelia burgdorferi* reaches the eye by hematogenous spread and may affect any ocular structure.[18–25] The main ocular findings in patients with Lyme disease consist of anterior uveitis, which could be granulomatous or nongranulomatous. Patients also may present with chronic cyclitis or pars planitis. Snowballs with peripheral vasculitis also may be seen. Vitreous cells and exudates may occur with involvement of the posterior segment. The posterior segment of the eye shows evidence of neuroretinitis with diffuse choroiditis involving and obliterating the choriocapillaris. Optic nerve hyperemia and edema also have been reported. Arterial hemorrhages also may be seen. Episcleritis, conjunctivitis, keratitis, iridocyclitis, retinal vasculitis, macular edema, pseudotumor cerebri, ischemic optic atrophy, and cranial nerve involvement have been seen. Inflammation of the choriocapillaris and retinal pigment epithelium may occur.[22] In severe cases, bilateral diffuse choroiditis with detachment of the retina may be observed.[26]

Laboratory Diagnosis

Gamma G immunoglobulin (IgG) and IgM antibodies to *Borrelia* may be determined by several tests, including monoclonal antibody indirect immunofluorescent technique and enzyme-linked immunosorbent assay (ELISA). The sensitivities of both serologic tests for Lyme disease are similar.

IgM antibodies are increased during the early phases of the disease. IgM antibodies may stay elevated in chronic cases for as long as 1 year. A false-positive test with low titer for syphilis may occur.

Treatment

The treatment of Lyme disease consists of the systemic administration of antibiotics for 3 weeks.[27] The treatment of acute systemic borreliosis without central nervous system or ocular involvement consists of the systemic administration of doxycycline 100 mg orally twice daily for 3 weeks or amoxicillin 500 mg orally four times daily for 3 weeks. Alternate therapy includes cefuroxime axetil 500 mg orally twice daily or azithromycin 500 mg orally daily for 7 days. The treatment of choice for Lyme disease with neuroretinitis and uveitis is the systemic administration of ceftriaxone 2 g IV daily for 14 days or penicillin G 20 million units IV per day for 14 to 21 days. Topical or subconjunctival steroids may be used in patients with severe intraocular inflammatory reactions. Topical mydriatic eyedrops should be used to prevent posterior synechiae.

Leptospirosis

Leptospirosis is a disease caused by *Leptospira icterohemorrhagiae*.

Clinical Findings

The predominant clinical findings in leptospirosis that follows Weil's disease is a bilateral, mild, nongranulomatous anterior uveitis.[28] The disease may be associated with focal choroiditis and retinal hemorrhages. Panuveitis may occur but it is rare.

Laboratory Diagnosis

Anterior chamber paracentesis may be performed, and aqueous humor specimen may yield useful results by agglutination in an attempt to measure the antibodies to leptospira.

Treatment

The treatment of choice for leptospirosis is the administration of oral doxycycline 100 mg orally twice a day for 21 days or amoxicillin 500 mg orally every 6 hours for 21 days.

References

1. Pace JL, Csonka GW: Endemic non-venereal syphilis (bejel) in Saudi Arabia. Br J Vener Dis 1984;60: 293–297.
2. Tabbara KF, Al-Kaff AS, Fadel T: Ocular manifestations of endemic syphilis (bejel). Ophthalmology 1989; 96(7):1087–1091.
3. Centers for Disease Control: Summary: cases of specified notifiable disease: United States. MMWR 1989; 37:802.
4. Tamesis RR, Foster CS: Ocular syphilis. Ophthalmology 1990;97:1281–1287.
5. Mancel E, Huet-Ernould F, Hugues P, et al.: Syphilitic uveitis. Bull Soc Ophthalmol Fr 1990;90(2): 199–204.
6. Friberg TR: Syphilitic chorioretinitis. Arch Ophthalmol 1989;107(11):1676–1677.
7. Zierhut M, Kreissig I, Pickert A: Panuveitis with positive serologic tests for syphilis and Lyme disease. J Clin Neuro Ophthalmol 1989;9(2):71–75.
8. Passo MS, Rosenbaum JT: Ocular syphilis in patients with human immunodeficiency virus infection. Am J Ophthalmol 1988;106:1–6.
9. Joyce PW, Haye KR, Ellis ME: Syphilitic retinitis in a homosexual man with concurrent HIV infection: Case report. Genitourin Med 1989;65(4):244–247.
10. Steere AC, Malawista SE, Syndman DR, et al.: Lyme arthritis: An epidemic of oligoarticular arthritis in children and adults in three Connecticut communities. Arthritis Rheum 1977;20:7–17.
11. Wallis RC, Brown SE, Kloter KO, et al.: Erythema chronicum migrans and Lyme arthritis: Field study of ticks. Am J Epidemiol 1978;108:222–227.
12. Spielman A, Clifford CM, Piesman J, et al.: Human babesiosis on Nantucket Island, USA: Description of the Vector, Ixodes dammini, n. sp. (Acarina: Ixodidae). J Med Entymol 1979;15:218–234.

13. Burgdorfer W, Barbour Ag, Hayes SF, et al.: Lyme disease: A tick-borne spirochetosis? Science 1982;216:1317–1319.
14. Schecter SL: Lyme disease associated with optic neuropathy. Am J Med 1986;81:143–145.
15. Schecter SL: Lyme disease associated with optic neuropathy. Am J Med 1986;81:143–145.
16. Steere AC, Malawista SE, Bartenhagen NH, et al.: The clinical spectrum and treatment of Lyme disease. Yale J Biol Med 1984;57:453–461.
17. Steere AC, Malawista SE, Hardin JA, et al.: Erythema chronicun migrans and Lyme arthritis: The enlarging spectrum. Ann Intern Med 1977;685–698.
18. Steere AC, Duray PH, Kauffman DJ, et al.: Unilateral blindness caused by infection with the Lyme disease spirochete Borrelia burgdorferi. Ann Intern Med 1985;103:382–384.
19. Winward KE, Smith JL, Culbertson WW, et al.: Ocular Lyme borreliosis. Am J Ophthalmol 1989:(6)I:651–677.
20. Kuiper H, Koelman JH, Jager MJ: Vitreous clouding associated with Lyme borreliosis. Am J Ophthalmol 1989;108:453–454.
21. Lesser RL, Kornmehl EW, Pachner AR, et al.: Neuro-ophthalmologic manifestations of Lyme disease. Ophthalmology 1990;97(6):699–706.
22. Bialasiewicz AA, Schonherr U: Choriocapillaritis (so-called pigment epithelitis) in Borrelia burgdorferi seroconversion. Klin Monatsbl Augenheilkd 1990;(6):481–483.
23. Oteo JA, Martinez de Artola V, Maravi E, et al.: Lyme disease and uveitis. Ann Intern Med 1990;122(11):883.
24. Baum J, Barza M, Weinstein P, et al.: Bilateral keratitis as a manifestation of Lyme disease. Am J Ophthalmol 1988;105:75–77.
25. Flach AJ, and Lavoie PE: Episcleritis conjunctivitis and keratitis as ocular manifestations of Lyme disease. Ophthalmology 1990;97:973–975.
26. Bialasiewicz AA, Ruprecht KW, Naumann GO, et al.: Bilateral diffuse choroiditis and exudative retinal detachments with evidence of Lyme disease. Am J Ophthalmol 1988;105:419–420.
27. Dattwyler RJ, Halperin JJ, Volkman DJ, et al.: Treatment of late Lyme Borreliosis: Randomized comparison of ceftriaxone penicillin. Lancet 1988;I:1191–1194.
28. Watt G: Leptospirosis as a cause of uveitis. Arch Intern Med 1990;150(5):1130–1132.

Mycobacterial Diseases

Tuberculosis

Tuberculosis is a chronic infection caused by the aerobic bacillus *Mycobacterium tuberculosis*. It is estimated that there are approximately 10 million new cases worldwide each year. The highest incidence of the disease occurs in Africa and Asia. It is also an important health problem in developed countries. The spread of human immunodeficiency virus (HIV) infection has recently increased the risk of tuberculosis in these countries.[1,2] In 1989 there was a total of 286 cases of new active tuberculosis in San Francisco, for a case rate of 38.9 cases per hundred thousand population. This is four times the provisional case rate of 9.1 per 100,000 in the United States. The World Health Organization (WHO) has estimated that at least five million people with HIV infection develop tuberculosis. The diagnosis of tuberculosis among patients with HIV infection may be difficult.[3,4]

Clinical Findings

Patients with pulmonary tuberculosis may not suffer from acute illness. Most of the symptoms are nonspecific, including chronic nonproductive cough in the early stages, which may become productive later. The cough may be associated with blood-streaked sputum and other nonspecific symptoms, including malaise, weight loss, fever, night sweat, anorexia, dyspepsia, excitement, and depression.

Ocular Findings of Tuberculosis

The ocular findings in patients with tuberculosis may occur with or without the presence of pulmonary findings. Patients develop anterior nongranulomatous or granulomatous uveitis. Patients who had been treated with topical steroid commonly present with nongranulomatous uveitis. The anterior inflammation of the eye is chronic and insidious. Posterior segment involvement leads to focal granuloma in the posterior pole or to multifocal choroiditis with overlying retinitis (Figures 4.6–4.10). The vitreous may show evidence of exudation and inflammatory cells. Focal areas of retinal vasculitis also may be seen in association with multifocal choroiditis. Most of the patients with vasculitis develop a phlebitis. The disease may be associated with a papillitis or optic neuritis and may cause decrease in vision.[5] Patients with HIV infection may develop geographic choroiditis.[6,12]

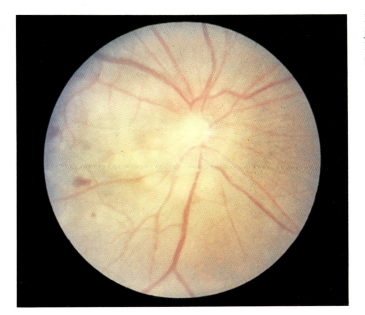

Figure 4.6. A 32-year-old man with active juxtapapillary tuberculous retinochoroiditis. Photo taken before initiation of systemic therapy.

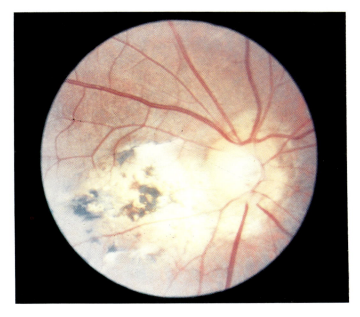

Figure 4.7. Same patient as in Figure 4.6 2 years after presentation and 1 year after a 1-year course with triple antituberculous therapy.

Diagnosis

The diagnosis of active pulmonary tuberculosis is achieved by either microscopic examination of sputum in smears or by culture. The bacilli are stained with acid-fast stain. Radiologic examination of the chest is essential for all patients with suspected tuberculosis. It should be emphasized, however, that negative chest radiograph does not rule out ocular tuberculosis. We had the opportunity to examine two patients with ocular tuberculosis who had no active pulmonary tuberculosis. In one patient who underwent enucleation, *Mycobacterium tuberculosis* was isolated from the ocular tissue and hematoxylin & eosin (H & E) stained sections showed multiple caseating granuloma. The chest radiograph on that patient was reported as normal.

The tuberculin skin test is important as an adjunct test in the diagnosis of tuberculosis. It consists of intradermal injection of purified protein

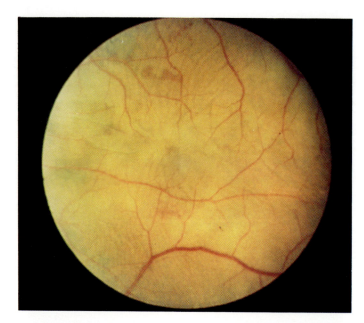

Figure 4.8. Tuberculous choroiditis.

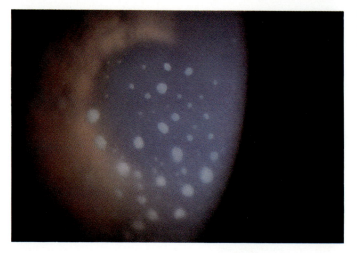

Figure 4.9. Anterior granulomatous uveitis in a patient with ocular tuberculosis and negative chest radiograph.

derivative of *mycobacterium tuberculosis* (PPD).[7] A total of 5 tuberculin units of PPD are injected intradermally. The reaction is read 48 to 72 hours after injection. A positive test indicated by the presence of induration of more than 10 mm (5 mm induration in patients with acquired immune deficiency syndrome [AIDS] is considered positive). False-positive results may occur in patients who had previous bacillus Calmette-Guerin (BCG) vaccination. If the test is negative, it may be repeated with a higher strength, such as 10 U PPD. In the pediatric age group, 1 U dose is advisable to start with. In patients with severe panuveitis, ocular fluids may be obtained, such as vitreous and aqueous.

The ocular fluids may be subjected to ELISA for the detection of mycobacterium antigen and antibody.[8] In addition, the vitreous specimen may be subjected to staining with acid-fast stain and culture for recovery of the *Mycobacterium tuberculosis* (Figures 4.11, 4.12). Recent new techniques for the diagnosis of tuberculosis have employed deoxyribonucleic acid (DNA) gene probes that hybridize Mycobacterial ribosomal ribonucleic acid (RNA) and are commercially available. The quantitative detection of adenosine deaminase in fluids (cerebrospinal fluid, pleural fluid), using colorimetric assay, have been used for diagnosis of tuberculosis. This is an enzyme of the purine salvage

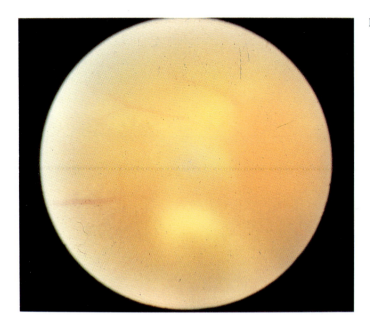

Figure 4.10. Tuberculous chorioretinitis.

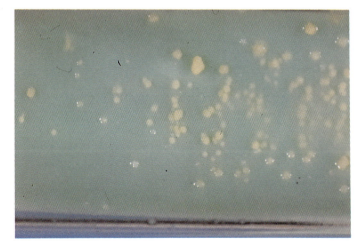

Figure 4.11. Hard dry creamy-white colonies of *Mycobacterium tuberculosis* isolated from eye of a patient with tuberculous chorioretinitis.

pathway whose main biologic role relates to the proliferation of lymphocytes with a higher specific activity in T lymphocytes than in B lymphocytes. Adenosine deaminase appears to be a sensitive marker for tuberculosis but has not been studied in ocular fluids.

We have found through a drug trial that isoniazid 300 mg orally per day for 2 weeks is not a good diagnostic test for ocular tuberculosis. We had one patient who was treated with isoniazid 300 mg orally for 3 weeks, and a vitreous specimen was obtained at that time. The patient showed no improvement in the ocular findings, and *Mycobacterium tuberculosis* was recovered from the vitreous specimen.

Treatment

Chemotherapeutic treatment of tuberculosis has changed over the past decade. Short-course chemotherapy of 6 months' duration using the four-drug combination of isoniazid, rifampicin, pyrazinamide, and ethambutol have been advocated for systemic tuberculosis (Table 4.1). It has been suggested to start the patient on the four-drug therapy, to discontinue the ethambutol after 2 months, and to continue with three-drug therapy for the remaining 4 months. This drug regimen has been found to be as effective as the standard 9-month daily course of therapy using isoniazid and rifampicin supplemented by ethambutol in the initial intensive

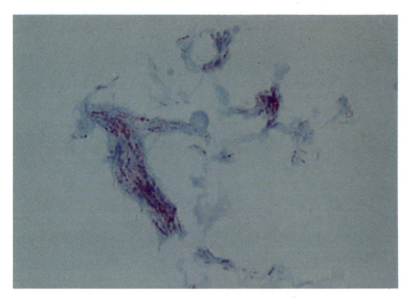

Figure 4.12. Acid-fast bacilli of *Mycobacterium tuberculosis.*

2-month phase. For ocular tuberculosis in adult patients, we have used the combination isoniazid 300 mg per day orally, rifampicin 600 mg per day orally, pyrazinamide 2 g per day orally, and ethambutol 800 mg per day. Pyridoxin 50 mg per day orally should be given to prevent isoniazid neurotoxicity. Ethambutol may be discontinued after 2 months of therapy. The treatment will have to be continued for 8 months. Adverse effects may occur, and several drugs may interact with antituberculous drugs (Table 4.2). The high cost of rifampicin may preclude its use in many developing countries.

It is estimated that 8% to 9% of *Mycobacterium tuberculosis* isolates are resistant to at least one drug.[9] The resistance to isoniazid is approximately 5%. It is always recommended to initiate patients with ocular tuberculosis on a minimum of the three-drug regimen.

Treatment of Patients with HIV Infection and Tuberculosis

Patients suffering from HIV infection and who are infected by *Mycobacterium tuberculosis* should be

Table 4.1. Drugs for Tuberculosis*

	Daily Doses (mg/kg)		Max. Daily Doses in Adults and Children	Frequency of Administration per Day
	Adults	Children		
Isoniazid[†] (p.o./IM)	5	10–20	300 mg	Single
Rifampicin (p.o.)	10	10–20	600 mg	Single
Pyrazinamide (p.o.)	20	15–30	2 g	3–4 divided doses
Ethambutol (p.o.)	15	15–25	2 g	Two doses
Streptomycin (IM)	15	20	1 g	Single

*p.o. = orally; IM = intramuscularly.
[†]Give supplemental pyridoxine 50 mg p.o. once daily.

Table 4.2. Adverse Effects of
Antituberculous Drugs

Drugs	Adverse Drug Reactions
Isoniazid	Hypersensitivity reaction fever, rash, urticaria. Hepatotoxicity, peripheral neuritis. Convulsions. Drug interactions: phenytoin, aluminum-containing antacids
Rifampin	Orange-pink discoloration of body fluids (sweat, tears, urine, saliva, milk, sputum, etc.). Gastrointestinal disturbances. Hypersensitivity reactions. Hematologic abnormalities: anemia and thrombocytopenia. Leukopenia. Hepatotoxicity. Drug interactions: warfarin, corticosteroids, oral contraceptives, sulphonylureas, diazepam, quinidine, methadone, and propranolol
Pyrazinamide	Hepatitis, hyperuricemia, nausea, vomiting, and drug fever
Ethambutol	Optic neuritis, hyperuricemia, skin rash
Streptomycin	Ototoxicity. Vestibular or auditory. Neuromuscular blockade, renal toxicity, hypersensitivity, skin rash, and fever.
Rifabutin	Hepatotoxicity, uveitis, fever, flushing pruritis, interstitial nephritis, orange color body fluids, thrombocytopenia. (Uveitis is common in patients under 55 kg of body weight.)
Clofazimine	Skin pigmentation, gastrointestinal intolerance

treated with the standard regimen as outlined in Table 4.1. In patients with atypical Mycobacterial infections, particularly *Mycobacterium avium complex*, the standard antituberculosis therapy is unsatisfactory, and a four-drug regimen including two other drugs—rifabutine and clofazimine—is recommended in the United States.[11] Recent studies have shown that the aminoglycoside, amikacin, and the quinolone, ciprofloxacin, may be used in combination with the antituberculous therapy.

Prophylaxis for Tuberculosis

Chemoprophylaxis may be indicated in patients who have uveitis attributable to immunologically mediated disorders and are found to be PPD positive. For chemoprophylaxis, patients may be given a two-drug therapy consisting of isoniazid and rifampicin.[10] The recommended treatment is a 3-month regimen of rifampicin and isoniazid. The treatment

has been shown to be safe and effective.[10] Resistance to therapy has been reported.[13] Most resistant cases occur in HIV-positive patients.

Rifabutine, a derivative of rifamycin, has been used in clinical trials for the treatment of tuberculosis in HIV-positive patients. Rifabutine, however, may cause uveitis in underweight individuals (< 55 kg in body weight).

Leprosy

Leprosy is a disease caused by *Mycobacterium leprae*. The disease may affect any structure of the eye, especially in the lepromatous form of the disease.

Clinical Findings

The eye is involved in 25% of patients with leprosy (Figures 4.13–4.16). Patients have involvement of the eye more commonly in the lepromatous form of the disease than in the tuberculoid or intermediate forms. Loss of hair of the lateral part of the eyebrow may be noted. Leonine facies is caused by involvement of the skin by the *Mycobacterium leprae*. Patients may develop cranial nerve involvement with keratitis. The involvement of the uvea is attributable to the lepromatous leprosy, in which case the anterior segment of the eye is more commonly affected than the posterior segment of the eye. This is because the organism prefers to proliferate in the cooler, exposed parts of the body. Massive localized granulomata of the iris and ciliary body may occur. Secondary glaucoma is common. Synechiae formation is seen, and cataract may occur. Lepromatous pearls are known to occur on the surface of the iris and may occur on the surface of the retina in aphakic patients. Leprosy, however, is not a primary disease of the retina and does not usually lead to choroiditis.[5]

Treatment

The treatment of leprosy consists of a combination of antimycobacterial antimicrobials. Patients with leprosy are given dapsone 100 mg orally per day, rifampin 600 mg orally per day, and clofazimine 100 mg orally per day. Topical therapy with steroids and antiglaucoma therapy (when indicated) are given for anterior uveitis.

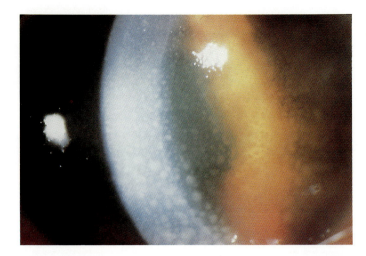

Figure 4.13. Anterior granulomatous uveitis in a patient with lepromatous leprosy.

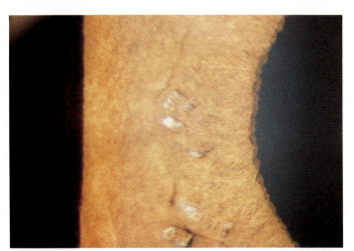

Figure 4.14. An "iris pearl" on the surface of the iris in a patient with leprosy.

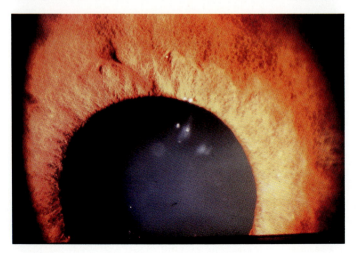

Figure 4.15. A case of leprosy with "iris pearl" at the pupillary border at the 1 o'clock position.

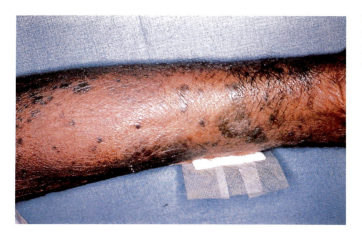

Figure 4.16. A patient with leprosy, showing involvement of the skin with areas of pigmentation. Skin biopsy was positive for *Mycobacterium leprae*.

References

1. Center for Disease Control: Tuberculosis in the US 1987. HHS Publication No. (CDC) 89-8322, 1989.
2. Bloch A, Rieder H, Kelly GD, et al.: The epidemiology of tuberculosis in the United States. Clin Chest Med 1989;10:297–313.
3. Watson J, Gill O: HIV infection and tuberculosis. Br Med J 1990;300:63–64.
4. Harries A: Tuberculosis and HIV infection in developing countries. Lancet 1990;335:387–390.
5. Kraus-Mackiw E, O'Connor GR: Uveitis: Pathophysiology and therapy. New York: George Thieme Verlag Stuttgart, 1986:63–64, 66–67.
6. Blodi BA, Johnson MW, McLeish WM, et al.: Presumed choroidal tuberculosis in a human immunodeficiency virus infected host. Am J Ophthalmol 1989;108(5):605–607.
7. Abrams J, Schlaegel TF: The tuberculin skin test in the diagnosis of tuberculous uveitis. Am J Ophthalmol 1983;96:295–298.
8. Watt G, Zaraspe G, Bautista S, Laughlin LW: Rapid diagnosis of tuberculosis meningitis by using an ELISA to detect mycobacterial antigen and antibody in cerebrospinal fluid. J Infect Dis 1988;158:681–686.
9. Iseman M, Madsen L: Drug resistant tuberculosis. Clin Chest Med 1989;10:341–353.
10. McNicol MW, Thomson H, Riordan JF, et al: Antituberculous chemoprophylaxis with isoniazid-rifampicin. Thorax 1984;39:223–224.
11. Center for Disease Control: US Department of Health and Human Services: Diagnosis and management of mycobacterial infection and disease in persons with HIV of mycobacterial infection and disease in persons with HIV infection. Ann Intern Med 1987; 106:254.
12. Blodi BA, Johnson MW, Mcleish WM, et al.: Presumed choroidal tuberculosis in a human immunodeficiency virus infected host. Am J Ophthalmol 1989;108(5):605–607.
13. Kim JY, Carroll CP, Opremcak, EM: Antibiotic-resistant tuberculous choroiditis (letter). Am J Ophthalmol 1993;115:259–261.

Other Bacterial Diseases

Brucellosis

Brucellosis is a zoonotic disease. Humans are accidental hosts playing little or no role in maintaining the disease or in the propagation of the organisms in nature. The disease is caused by a gram-negative bacterium known as *Brucella*. There are four main species of brucella that may cause disease in man: *Brucella melitensis, Brucella abortus, Brucella suis,* and *Brucella canis. Brucella melitensis* and *Brucella abortus* are the most common organisms causing brucellosis in humans.[1] The disease has been controlled in Western countries but remains endemic in many developing countries. Sgt. Major David Bruce discovered the organism on December 26, 1886 in Malta, after performing an autopsy on a young private soldier. He named the organism *Micrococcus melitensis,* and it was later designated by the term brucella after David Bruce. The disease is referred to as Mediterranean, Malta, or undulant fever.

Epidemiology

The disease is transmitted to humans through the ingestion of unpasteurized milk and milk products or the ingestion of uncooked meat. Brucellosis is also known to be an occupational hazard for laboratory workers, veterinarians, farmers, and shepherds, as well as meat inspectors. Airborne spread of brucellosis has been reported.[2] The disease has a worldwide distribution, but is under control in Scandinavian and Western countries. The disease is still endemic in many developing countries and remains a public health problem. Brucellosis is considered to be among those zoonotic disorders with significant impact on human health. Brucella was in fact first isolated from humans despite the fact that the disease has been known to cause contagious abortion in goats, cattle, and swine since the turn of the century. Milk from diseased animals continues to be the chief source of human infection despite efforts in many countries to eradicate the disease. Although brucellosis is an uncommon infection in developed countries, there is always the danger that tourists and other travelers may become infected abroad and, on their return to their home country, they may develop symptoms of the illness.[3] At that stage the early diagnosis of brucellosis may be missed. In the United States, the incidence of human brucellosis declined dramatically after the enforcement of laws requiring pasteurization of milk and the adoption of uniform rules set forth in the bovine brucellosis eradication program of the Department of Agriculture. Brucellosis control is a financial burden and requires large-scale testing of cattle to detect serologically positive animals. In addition, such campaigns require the administration of vaccines to immature heifers using brucella strain 19. Infected animals are slaughtered. In the United States, cattle infected with *Brucella abortus* have been the major natural reservoir of brucellosis. The number of human cases of brucellosis in the United States is fewer than 100 per year, compared with 10% of the population among certain communities of countries in the Middle East. Two outbreaks of human brucellosis caused by *Brucella melitensis* occurred in Texas in 1985. The source of infection was traced to unpasteurized goat cheese made in Mexico. Goat's milk cheese is traditionally eaten within a few days of production to preserve its distinctive flavor. Pasteurization is claimed to result in an inferior product. For this reason, several types of cheese produced in many countries use unpasteurized milk.

Brucella are killed in the laboratory by heating at 60°C for 10 minutes or by 10% phenol for 15 minutes. In cow sheds, the organisms may survive for many months, and in animal feces at 8°C they may survive for more than 1 year. The brucella organism may persist in milk for several days, but when the milk turns sour the acidity may kill the organism. Brucella in the cow infects the placenta and vaginal discharges after delivery or abortion. Cows may lick these products and may ingest brucella, spreading the organism and the disease. The organism may spread heavily in the environment and may be inhaled or enter the animal through the conjunctival sac. In Saudi Arabia, cows, sheep, goats, and camels may be infected with brucella. Adults taking antacids are more susceptible to brucella because gastric acidity may kill the organism. Person-to-person spread is rare but has been reported. Grave and Sturm[4] reported an outbreak of brucellosis associated with the use of bovine placental extracts and fetal cells in a beauty parlor. The preparation is known as "la biogenese hibernee," which was used in beauty parlors in Holland by rubbing on the patient's skin as a cosmetic.

Clinical Findings

The most characteristic finding of brucellosis is undulating fever. Fever occurs in many ways; patients with brucellosis complain of malaise, anorexia, night sweating, headache, and generalized aches and pains. The initial acute phase of the disease may go into spontaneous remissions or exacerbations or may become chronic and last for many years. Patients with chronic brucellosis may develop complications such as arthritis. The joints involved are usually unilateral and peripheral, most commonly affecting the hip or knee. Spondylitis also may occur leading to paravertebral abscess. Other complications include endocarditis with involvement of the heart valves. Brucella pericarditis and myocarditis also have been reported. Pulmonary brucellosis may occur, and neurologic complications are common.

Inflammations of the retina and uvea may occur in brucellosis.[5] The ocular involvement may be mild, with anterior uveitis or it may be severe, with panophthalmitis (Figure 4.17). The anterior uveitis

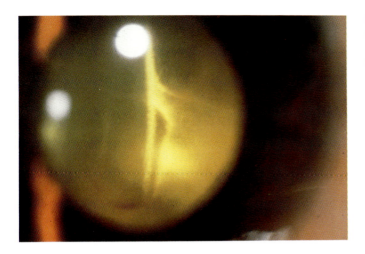

Figure 4.17. A 36-year-old male with ocular brucellosis, showing fibrinous exudates in the vitreous. *Brucella melitensis* was isolated from the eye.

may be granulomatous or non-granulomatous and patients may develop vitreitis. A hypopyon may occur, which may disappear spontaneously without treatment in 3 to 4 days. Scleritis also may occur in patients with brucellosis and should be differentiated from other rheumatic diseases that may lead to scleritis and uveitis. Retinal vasculitis may occur. The most characteristic finding of posterior uveitis is a geographic choroiditis, which occurred in three of five patients who suffered from ocular brucellosis.[5] Optic neuritis has been reported. Patients may develop extensive vitreous.[6] In certain untreated cases, panuveitis may occur. Occasionally, patients may present with intermediate uveitis.[7]

Laboratory Diagnosis

The standard test for brucellosis is the agglutination test. The test is performed in increasing dilutions to prevent blocking of antibodies that may be present. IgG and IgM antibodies to brucella may be determined. Complement fixation test is also available for the diagnosis of brucella. Recently, an enzyme immunoassay incorporating a *Brucella militensis* outer membrane protein antigen has been successful in confirming infection with the common *Brucella* species. A radioimmunoassay measuring brucella IgM and IgG can improve the sensitivity and specificity of serologic testing. Isolation of the organism from the ocular fluid may be achieved by obtaining vitreous specimens. Antibodies to brucella may be detected in the aqueous

and vitreous fluid. The organism may be isolated from aqueous or vitreous.

Treatment

Rifampin 600 mg orally per day with doxycycline 200 mg orally per day is considered to be the treatment of choice. The treatment may be prescribed for a period of 6 to 8 weeks. Intramuscular injection of streptomycin also may be used. Recently, a third-generation cephalosporin, ceftriaxone or ceftizoxime, have been shown to have remarkable bactericidal activity to *Brucella melitensis*.[8]

In conclusion, brucellosis remains to be a public health problem in several areas of the world. Early detection of this condition and prompt treatment may lead to full recovery and complete cure. Although autoimmune or other immunologically mediated disorders afflicting the posterior segment of the eye may respond to treatment with systemic and topical immunosuppressive agents, such therapy may prove to be devastating in cases of infectious origin affecting the posterior segment of the eye. Although certain infections affecting the posterior segment of the eye, such as brucellosis, are more endemic in certain regimens of the world, air travel and tourism are breaking these geographic barriers.

Pathology

The invasion of tissues by brucella leads to focal granuloma formation, and the pathologic lesions are caused by the proliferation of bacterial organism within the tissues. The vasculitis in patients with brucellosis is probably caused by the deposition of immune complexes in the vessel wall. The typical histopathologic lesion consists of chronic, non-specific inflammation characterized by the presence of lymphocytes, plasma cells, and occasional polymorphonuclear cells and histocytes and scattered granulomas composed of epithelioid cells, but no central caseation is seen.

Nocardiosis

Nocardiosis is a disease caused by *Nocardia asteroides*. *Nocardia* is a ubiquitous bacterium found in soil. The disease is acquired by inhalation or in-gestion of the organism. Nocardiosis is a rare disease that afflicts debilitated or immunosuppressed individuals.

Clinical Findings

The eye may be involved after a systemic infection. The systemic infection may be subclinical, and the ocular findings could be the initial presenting manifestation of the disease (Figures 4.18, 4.19). Patients with systemic nocardiosis may have chronic lung disease or pneumonia, liver abscess, or sometimes brain abscess. The posterior segment of the eye may be involved in nocardiosis. The characteristic finding is a focal choroidal infiltration with a retinal necrosis and detachment. The vitreous may show evidence of inflammatory changes.

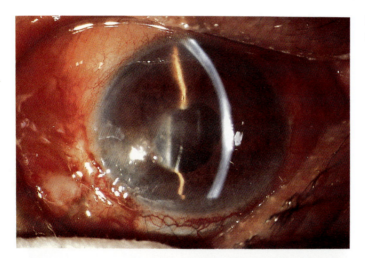

Figure 4.18. An 80-year-old man with *Nocardia* scleritis and intraocular invasion.

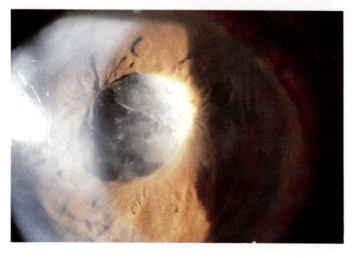

Figure 4.19. Same patient shown in Figure 4.18. Fibrinous clot behind the iris secondary to intraocular spread of *Nocardia*.

The diagnosis of nocardiosis is confirmed by the isolation of the organism from the vitreous or by an eye wall biopsy.

Treatment

Treatment of nocardiosis consists of systemic administration of antimicrobial agents such as trimethoprim 15 mg/kg with sulfamethoxazole 75 mg/kg daily in three doses or minocycline 100 mg orally twice daily for 2 days and then 100 mg orally per day for 3 weeks.

Meningococcosis

Meningococcosis is a disease caused by *Neisseria meningitidis*. The disease is uncommon, and the most frequently encountered clinical finding is meningitis. Early diagnosis and prompt treatment are essential and may be life saving.

Clinical Findings

Patients develop meningococcemia with skin rashes that show purpuric lesions. Patients develop fever, headache, and signs of meningitis.

The main ocular findings consist of anterior nongranulomatous uveitis associated with ciliary injection and photophobia. Patients develop exudations in the vitreous. The infection may reach the eye through the optic nerve head in cases of meningitis. Juxtapapillary retinitis and choroiditis are seen in patients with meningitis. Posterior segment lesions also may appear as focal retinitis. Patients may develop endogenous meningococcal endophthalmitis with vitreous exudates.

Laboratory Diagnosis

Blood should be subjected to cultures. It should be performed in patients suspected of having meningococcal infections. Culture of vitreous specimens is done in cases with vitritis.

Treatment

Treatment of meningococcal infection consists of the systemic administration of a third-generation cephalosporin: cefotaxime, ceftriaxone, or ceftizomine, ampicillin, or penicillin may be added for older patients (>18 years of age).

References

1. Young EJ: Human brucellosis. Rev Infect Dis 1983; 5(5):821–842.
2. Kaufmann AF, Fox MD, Anderson DC, et al.: Airborne spread of brucellosis. Ann NY Sci 1980;353:105–114.
3. Steffen R: Antacids: A risk factor in traveller's brucellosis. Scand J Infect Dis 1977;9:311–312.
4. Grave W, Sturm AW: Brucellosis associated with a beauty parlour. Lancet 1983;1:1326–1327.
5. Tabbara KF, Al-Kassimi H: Ocular brucellosis. Br J Ophthalmol 1990;74(4):249–250.
6. Tabbara KF: Brucellosis and endemic syphilis. Int Ophthalmol Clin 1990;30;294–296.
7. Lepori JC, Briquel F, Gerar A, Reny A: Pars planite et brucellose. Ann Med Nancy Est 1982;21:565–570.
8. Palenque E, Otero JR, Noriega Ar: In-vitro susceptibility of Brucella malitensis to new cephalosporins crossing the blood brain barrier. Antimicrob Agents Chemother 1986:29:182–183.

Chapter 5
Parasitic Infections

Khalid F. Tabbara and Aniki Rothova*

Toxoplasmosis

Ocular toxoplasmosis is a common infection of the retina and choroid caused by the parasite: *Toxoplasma gondii*. The initial ocular infection may follow a systemic infection *in utero* or later in life. The initial lesion appears as a focal infection in the retina. The disease recurs in the eye without systemic manifestations and can cause relentless damage to the retina or other structures of the posterior segment of the eye. Acute toxoplasmic retinochoroiditis has been generally regarded as a late manifestation of congenital toxoplasmosis. Over the past few years, however, we have seen an increasing number of cases with ocular lesions that follow acquired systemic toxoplasmosis. Ocular lesions as a manifestation of an initial acquired systemic toxoplasmosis have been reported.[1,2] Ocular toxoplasmosis may follow acquired systemic toxoplasmosis. The onset of toxoplasmic retinochoroiditis may occur concomitantly, immediately after, or years after the systemic illness. Several family members may also be affected.[3]

Epidemiology

Humans can acquire toxoplasmosis in any of three ways:

1. Ingestion of oocysts: Oocysts of *Toxoplasma* are shed in cat feces deposited in sandboxes and soil around homes, barnyards, and fields.[4] Contamination of vegetables and accidental contamination of hands may facilitate ingestion of oocysts.
2. Ingestion of toxoplasma bradyzoites or the encysted form of the parasite in undercooked meat (pork, beef, mutton, chicken). The encysted form of the parasite has been shown to persist in the flesh of many animals used for domestic meat production.
3. Tachyzoites (the proliferative form of the parasite): Women with no immunity to toxoplasma organisms may acquire toxoplasmosis during pregnancy and transmit the disease to the fetus by transplacental transmission of the tachyzoites. Laboratory personnel working with *T. gondii* occasionally may acquire the disease by accidental inoculation of the tachyzoites by skin penetration with infected needles. After parasitemia, the organisms can enter all types of cells, commonly the brain, eyes, striated muscles, and reticuloendothelial system.
4. By organ transplantation (rare): Ryning and co-workers[5] reported two heart transplant recipients who developed toxoplasmosis shortly after surgery.

*The section on Onchocerciasis (starting on page 65) is written by Aniki Rothova whose affiliations are the Department of Ophthalmology, Academic Medical Centre, Amsterdam, and Department of Ophthalmo-Immunology, The Netherlands Ophthalmic Research Institute, Amsterdam, The Netherlands.

Table 5.1. Ocular Toxoplasmosis

Definition

Ocular toxoplasmosis is a common infection of the retina and is caused by an obligate intracellular parasite known as *Toxoplasma gondii*. The initial ocular infection may be acquired *in utero* or later in life and represents a focal infection in the retina following parasitemia.

I. Clinical Presentation
  A. Symptoms
    1. Sudden onset of floating spots
    2. Blurring or haziness of vision
    3. Rarely pain, redness, and photophobia
  B. Cardinal Signs
    1. Yellow-white lesion on the retina with fuzzy borders
    2. Pigmented atrophic retinochoroiditic scar adjacent and contiguous to the lesion or elsewhere in the fundus
    3. Vitreous cells, strands, or precipitates on the posterior hyaloid
    4. Focal areas of vasculitis in the vicinity of the lesion that sometimes appear like beading of blood vessels, which may affect either the vein or artery
    5. Edema of the retina and sometimes macular edema, particularly if the lesion occurs superior to the macula
    6. Hyperemia and edema of the optic nerve head with congestion of veins
  C. Anterior Segment Signs
    1. Cells and flare in the anterior chamber in an otherwise quiet eye, or variable amounts of cells and flare in the anterior chamber
    2. KPs, which may appear either fine or mutton-fat
    3. Hyperemia of the iris
    4. Other findings: in recurrent cases, such as posterior synechiae, complicated cataract, and glaucoma
II. Laboratory Tests
  A. Blood tests: "Toxoplasma dye test" may be positive at the very low titer. Other blood tests include hemagglutination test and ELISA. The indirect fluorescent antibody test may be performed for the detection of IgG, IGA, and IgM. IgM antibodies are elevated in acute acquired systemic disease.
  B. Tests of limited usefulness, complement fixation tests, and precipitating antibody tests.
  C. Tests of ocular fluids, antibody levels in the aqueous and vitreous can be determined by the ELISA. Toxoplasma antigens in the aqueous or vitreous also may be detected by the ELISA.
  D. X-ray of the skull in patients with suspected congenital toxoplasmosis may show calcification.
  E. Polymerase chain reaction
III. Treatment
  A. Pyrimethamine 75 mg per day for 2 consecutive days. Then pyrimethamine 25 mg per day for 6 weeks thereafter. Complete blood count and platelet count should be performed while patient is on pyrimethamine. Sulfonamides, sulfadiazine, or triple sulfa (2 g orally stat, followed by 0.5 g four times daily for 6 weeks).
       Folinic acid 3 mg intramuscularly or orally twice a week as required. Force fluids and give patient sodium bicarbonate 1 teaspoonful three times per day to alkalinize the urine and prevent crystallization of sulfa in the renal tubules.
  B. Clindamycin 300 mg orally every 6 hours for 4 weeks, combined with pyrimethamine as mentioned above.
  C. Azithromycin (Pfizer) 500 mg orally once a day for 3 to 4 weeks (investigational).
  D. Atovaquone (Burroughs Wellcome) 750 mg p.o. three times daily (investigational).
  E. Indication for the use of systemic corticosteroid dosage, 80 to 100 mg per day in four divided doses for 1 week, then tapered over the next 8 weeks. Do not give periocular injections of depo corticosteroids.
    1. Paramacular lesion
    2. Vision-threatening papillomacular bundle involvement
    3. Optic nerve lesions or juxtapapillary lesions
    4. Massive vitreous reaction without detachment of the hyaloid face
  F. Photocoagulation and cryotherapy rarely indicated.

Clinical Findings

Acquired systemic toxoplasmosis is common and is frequently a subclinical infection (Table 5.1). Systemic toxoplasmosis is characterized by fever associated with maculopapular rash and benign lymphadenopathy. The disease may resemble rubella and infectious mononucleosis. Ocular in-

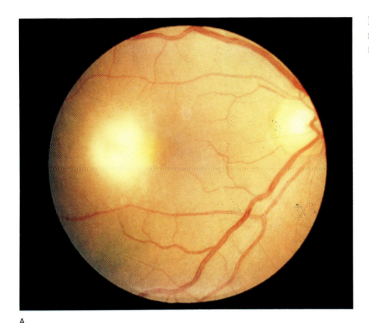

A

Figure 5.1. A. Focus of acute necrotizing retinitis in a patient with ocular toxoplasmosis. **B.** Close-up view of the same lesion.

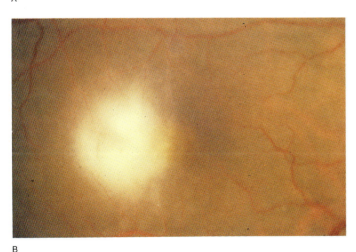

B

volvement in the course of acquired systemic toxoplasmosis is common.[3] The incidence of retinochoroiditis in patients with systemic toxoplasmosis is difficult to determine because of the asymptomatic nature of the infection in most cases.

Congenital toxoplasmosis, however, presents a variety of clinical pictures that range from a mild subclinical disease to a fulminant infection with a fatal outcome. The disease may affect the central nervous system. Bilateral retinochoroiditis is the most common feature of the disease, occurring in 86% to 96% of the cases. Other features of congenital toxoplasmosis are abnormal cerebrospinal fluid,

hepatosplenomegaly, anemia, jaundice, convulsions, and intracranial calcifications. Infants may develop a macular skin rash, lymphadenopathy, vomiting, pneumonia, and diarrhea.

Ocular toxoplasmosis begins as a focal area of necrotizing retinochoroiditis surrounded by retinal edema (Figure 5.1). The active lesion is often seen at the border or contiguous with old retinochoroiditis scars (Figures 5.2, 5.3). Toxoplasmic retinochoroiditis may be a single lesion or multiple foci that can be small or several disk diameters in size. Punched-out lesions with varying amounts of pigments in or around them may be seen (Figures

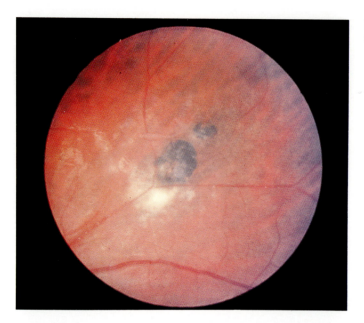

Figure 5.2. A small area of retinitis adjacent to a toxoplasmic retinochoroiditic scar.

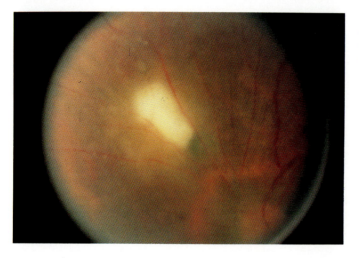

Figure 5.3. Active toxoplasmic retinochoroiditis lesion. Note the small pigmented scar inferior to the active retinochoroiditis lesion.

5.4–5.6). The average duration of the natural course of ocular toxoplasmosis in uncompromised hosts may last up to 10 weeks. In rare instances, a lesion may last longer. Healing is associated with sharpening of the borders, decrease in retinal edema, and development of pigmentary changes or clumps of pigment at the borders of these lesions. Retinal vasculitis, which could be phlebitis or arteritis, frequently may occur in association with toxoplasmic retinochoroiditis. Vasculitis leads to vascular occlusion, resulting in retinal hemorrhages. Loss of visual acuity in ocular toxoplasmosis may be caused by the vitreous opacities, cystoid macular edema, or inflammatory foci in the macula, papillomacular bundle, or optic nerve. Anterior uveitis is associated with toxoplasmic retinochoroiditis. The iris and ciliary body can be affected by an intense inflammation, which may cause marked ciliary injection, keratitis precipitates, flare and cells in the aqueous humor, nodules on the iris, and posterior synechiae. The uveitis may be severe enough to cause an increase in intraocular pressure. Recurrence of toxoplasmic retinochoroiditis is common in areas adjacent to healed retinochoroiditic scars. These scars have been shown to contain *Toxoplasma* cysts containing viable bradyzoites (Figure

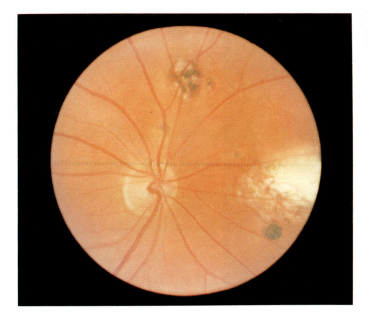

Figure 5.4. Healed multiple toxoplasmic retinochoroiditic scars in a patient with bilateral congenital ocular toxoplasmosis.

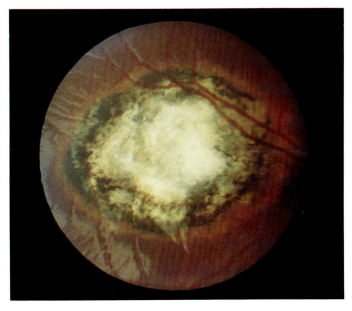

Figure 5.5. Punched-out toxoplasmic retinochoroiditic scar.

5.7). When the cyst wall breaks down from any one of a number of causes, bradyzoites escape and the organisms are transformed into tachyzoites that soon invade neighboring cells, leading to tissue destruction (see Figure 5.8).

Laboratory Investigations

Toxoplasma antibodies can be detected by various serologic techniques, including Sabin-Feldman dye test, the indirect fluorescent antibody test, the hemagglutination test, the precipitant test, and enzyme-linked immunosorbent assay (ELISA). A positive test is considered to be significant when the ocular lesion is compatible with toxoplasmosis. Recurrences of ocular toxoplasmosis are usually not associated with an increase in antibody titers. The level of *Toxoplasma* antibody titer, moreover, seems not to be related to the activity of the ocular disease. Systemic infection with *Toxoplasma* organisms,

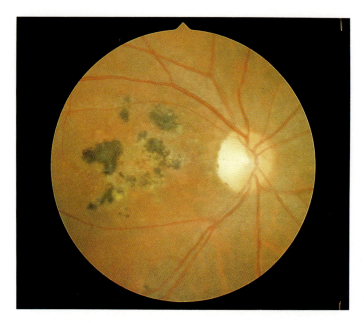

Figure 5.6. Pigmented toxoplasmic scars of the retina.

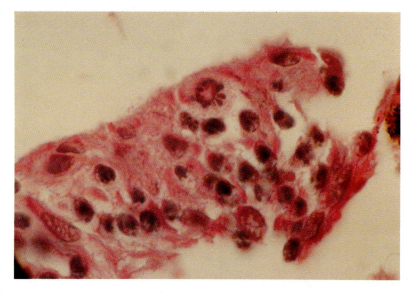

Figure 5.7. Cyst of *Toxoplasma gondii* in the retina of a rabbit with experimental ocular toxoplasmosis.

however, is associated with high serum antibody titers. *Toxoplasma* antibodies and antigens can be detected in the aqueous humor by the ELISA. Polymerase chain reaction has been used for the detection of toxoplasma antigens in ocular tissues.[6] IgA antitoxoplasma antibodies are specifically elevated in congenital toxoplasmosis.

Treatment

Various therapeutic regimens have been recommended for ocular toxoplasmosis.[7–13] The treatment of toxoplasmic retinochoroiditis in AIDS requires a long-term course with antimicrobial agents.

Pyrimethamine and sulfa can be administered singly or in combination. The drugs have been extensively investigated in both animals and humans. Pyrimethamine and sulfonamides act synergistically to inhibit folic acid synthesis. In immunocompetent hosts small lesions in the periphery of the retina with no significant vitreous cells can be observed clinically without treatment. Treatment of larger lesions of toxoplasma retinochoroiditis consists of giving a loading dose of pyrimethamine, 75 mg orally, followed by 25 mg orally daily for 4 to 6 weeks. This therapy can be combined with sulfonamides, 2 g as a loading dose, followed by 0.5 g four times daily for 4 to 6 weeks. The urine should be kept slightly alkaline by advising the patient to take one teaspoonful of sodium bicarbonate with each meal and to take fluids. Folinic acid supplementation is indicated to prevent bone marrow depression, characterized by leukopenia and thrombocytopenia. Folinic acid in 3-mg ampules can be mixed with fruit juice and given to the patient orally twice a week. An economical and effective substitute for folinic acid is brewer's yeast. Patients receiving pyrimethamine can be advised to take 1 tablespoonful of brewer's yeast three times per day. Treatment of certain large lesions of toxoplasmic retinochoroiditis with pyrimethamine and sulfonamides has produced unpredictable and sometimes disappointing clinical results. Frequent monitoring of hematopoietic function is essential. Leukocyte and platelet counts should be monitored at least once a week. One may elect to observe clinically small retinal lesions less than 0.25 disc diameter in size and located in the periphery of the retina with mild or no vitreous reaction.

In congenital toxoplasmosis associated with active retinochoroiditis, give pyrimethamine, 1 mg/kg/24 hours at 12-hour intervals to a maximum dose of 25 mg per day. After 4 days, the dose should be reduced to 0.5 mg/kg/24 hours and maintained at this level for 4 weeks. Bone marrow depression is dose-related, and platelet and white counts should be tested every other day. Treatment of affected infants should be given in the hospital. Pyrimethamine can be combined with sulfadiazine in a concentration of 100 to 150 mg/kg/24 hours. The combined drugs are given orally in four divided doses for 4 weeks. Folinic acid should be given as a single daily dose of 1 mg/kg/24 hours. It is essential to monitor the hematopoietic function.

In recent studies, the author and others[8,9] have shown that treatment of toxoplasmic retinochoroiditis with clindamycin, alone or in combination with sulfadiazine, induced healing. Clindamycin can be given orally, 300 mg four times per day for 4 to 6 weeks. This may be combined with sulfadiazine, 4 gm daily in four divided doses. The higher ocular absorption of clindamycin,[9] its possible penetration of the *Toxoplasma* cysts,[10] and its apparent efficacy in the treatment of acute toxoplasmic retinochoroiditis are strongly in its favor as a therapeutic alternative to pyrimethamine and sulfonamides. Clindamycin can be reserved for patients who cannot tolerate pyrimethamine or who show no response to combined therapy with pyrimethamine and sulfonamides. About 10% to 15% of patients treated with clindamycin develop pseudomembranous colitis, which is felt to be due to the proliferation of a clindamycin-resistant organism, *Clostridium difficile*. This condition is reversible upon discontinuing clindamycin and administration of oral vancomycin.

Trimethoprim-sulfamethoxazole may be given as prophylactic therapy in patients with AIDS.

Minocycline is a semisynthetic tetracycline analog that acts by inhibiting microbial protein synthesis. The drug has a broad spectrum of antibacterial activity and is effective in a treatment of infection with chloroquine-resistant *Plasmodium falciparum*. In a murine model of toxoplasmosis, we have shown that minocycyline was effective in eradicating the organism and ameliorating the course of the disease. In the murine model of toxoplasmosis, minocycline was found to be effective (P = .001) in the treatment of the disease and appeared to have a synergistic action with sulfadiazine. We studied the effects of minocycline on experimentally induced toxoplasmic retinochoroiditis in the rabbit. In a series of experiments, we found the drug effective in ameliorating the clinical disease and eradicating *Toxoplasma* organisms from the ocular tissues.[11]

Investigational drug (566C 80) atovaquone hydroxynaphthaquinone, an antimalarial agent, has been used successfully in the treatment of toxoplasmic retinochoroiditis in patients with AIDS.[13a] Atovaquone is available from Burroughs Wellcome. The recommended dose is 750 mg p.o. three times daily. New macrolides such as azithromycin have also been shown to be effective in the treatment of toxoplasmosis. A combination of atovaquone, azithromycin, and pyrimethamine has been used for the treatment of cerebral toxoplasmosis in patients with AIDS.

Topical corticosteroids may reduce the hypersensitivity reaction in the anterior segment of the eye. In nonhuman primates, the severity of anterior uveitis can be correlated with the number of organisms injected in the posterior segment of the eye. The anterior uveitis, therefore, is believed to be a result of a hypersensitivity reaction. For this purpose, a local corticosteroid such as prednisolone, 1% eye-drops, can be used four to five times per day as indicated in combination with a topical mydriatic agent such as cyclopentolate 1%, or tropicamide 1%, one drop twice daily.

Recurrence of ocular toxoplasmosis is thought to be caused by proliferation of the parasite and hypersensitivity reactions in retinal tissue. Toxoplasmic retinal infection induces an exudative inflammatory reaction that can lead to eradication of the parasite. This reaction, however, can lead also to retinal damage.

Although corticosteroids effectively quell the inflammatory reactions and partly prevent the tissue damage, at the same time, they suppress immune defense mechanisms. This leads to proliferation of the parasite and causes chronic, relentless destruction of the ocular structures. The risk/benefit ratio should be carefully assessed. The use of systemic corticosteroids can be justified when vision is seriously threatened; for example (1) lesions close to or in the macular area; (2) juxtapapillary lesions; such as lesions close to the optic nerve head; (3) large, granulomas with extensive vitreous reaction; (4) cystoid macular edema; and (5) lesions occupying the papillomacular bundle or lesions associated with extensive retinal vasculitis. Corticosteroids should always be used with appropriate antimicrobial therapy as previously outlined. They should never be used alone and should not be used at all if visual function is not threatened. When corticosteroids must be used, give prednisone, 80 to 100 mg daily orally (or equivalent) for 1 to 2 weeks and taper downward over 2 to 3 weeks. Periocular injections of corticosteroids should not be considered in ocular toxoplasmosis because this would deliver high levels of the drug to the ocular lesion, and in cases of long-acting corticosteroids would lead to unrestricted proliferation of the organisms because of suppression of the defense mechanisms.[15]

To determine the current practices in the management of ocular toxoplasmosis, 72 of 85 ophthalmologists of the American Uveitis Society completed a detailed questionnaire.[12] Ophthalmologists treat an average of ten patients for ocular toxoplasmosis per year. The antimicrobial agents are used and tailored based on the ocular findings. Approximately two-thirds of the ophthalmologists do not treat if vision is 20/20 and the lesion is peripheral. The preferred therapeutic regimens for typical

ocular toxoplasmosis by members of the American Uveitis Society are shown in Table 5.2.

Prevention of toxoplasmosis may be achieved by avoiding the consumption of undercooked meat including chicken, beef, mutton, and pork. Children should not be allowed to play in sand or soil contaminated with cat feces. Pregnant women who are toxoplasma antibody negative should avoid contact with cats. Furthermore, routine neonatal screening for toxoplasmosis identifies cases of subclinical congenital infection, and early treatment of such cases may reduce the severe long-term sequalae of toxoplasmosis.[14] Infected newborns may not show clinical manifestations of the disease at birth but by age 20 the majority will develop toxoplasmic retinochoroiditis.[15]

Trypanosomiasis

Trypanosomiasis is caused by *Trypanosoma gambiense* and *Trypanosoma rhodesiense*. At the time of parasitemia, the protozoa may reach the ocular structures, leading to uveitis.[16]

Clinical Findings

Trypanosomiasis may lead to hemorrhagic retinitis and iridocyclitis. It was produced in sheep by intravenous inoculation of *Trypanosoma brucei*.

Table 5.2. Therapeutic Regimens (1990) For Typical Cases* of Ocular Toxoplasmosis

Drug Combination	Responding Ophthalmologists
Pyrimethamine/folinic acid, sulfadiazine, and prednisone	32% (20/62)
Pyrimethamine/folinic acid, sulfadiazine, Clindamycin, and prednisone	27% (17/62)
Clindamycin, prednisone, with or without sulfadiazine	22% (14/62)

*A typical case was defined as an immunocompetent patient with a macular or optic nerve, head-threatening lesion, who was decreased central vision, but had potential for full recovery of central vision (Pregnant females were excluded). Modified from Engstrom RE, Holland GN, Nussenblatt RB, and Jabs DA: Current practices in the management of ocular toxoplasmosis. Am J Ophthalmol 1991;111:601.

Amoebiasis

Clinical Findings

The presence of focal central choroiditis associated with macular edema has been reported in patients suffering from *Entamoeba histolytica* enteritis. The diagnosis of amoebiasis of the choroid is circumstantial and has not been confirmed by isolation of the organism from ocular tissue.

Hartmanella and *Acanthamoeba* may produce retinal choroiditis and optic neuritis in experimental animals. *Acanthamoeba* may produce meningoencephalitis.

Toxocariasis

Toxocariasis is a parasitic disease caused by the larva forms of the roundworm *Toxocara canis.*

Clinical Findings

The ocular form of toxocariasis is attributed to the presence of the larva of the parasite in ocular tissues. The major ocular manifestations of toxocariasis in humans include: (1) a localized granuloma of the posterior segment of the eye, (2) a focal chronic inflammation of the retinal periphery simulating chronic cyclitis or pars planitis, and (3) diffuse panuveitis with endophthalmitis. The disease affects children and young adults and appears to be caused by the ingestion of toxocara eggs. Visceral larva migrans is a systemic form of toxocariasis occurring in children younger than 5 years of age and associated with febrile lymphadenopathy, hepatosplenomegaly, and eosinophilia. Ocular lesions are rare in visceral larva migrans. Table 5.3 demonstrates the difference between ocular larva migrans and visceral larva migrans.

The posterior segment involvement of ocular toxocariasis shows a posterior pole elevated mound of tissue in the area of localized granuloma in or around the macular area (Figure 5.8). The lesion may be accompanied by focal hemorrhages or serous detachment of the retina. The lesion may simulate retinoblastoma or endophthalmitis. Scarring and contraction of the ocular tissue may lead to the dragging of the optic nerve head toward the temporal periphery (Figure 5.9). Hogan and associates found a larval worm in the snowbank exudates that was seen in the inferior pars plana region of a patient who suffered from ocular toxocariasis which was previously diagnosed as chronic cyclitis or pars planitis. Ocular toxocariasis may simulate pars planitis or intermediate uveitis. Other clinical manifestations may include hypopyon, motile larva in vitreous, optic neuritis, and vitreous abscess.

Laboratory Diagnosis

Ocular toxocariasis may be confirmed by testing aqueous or vitreous specimens as well as serum for the presence of gamma G immunoglobulin (IgG) and IgE antibodies to *Toxocara*. The antibody titers in the vitreous may appear to be higher than the serum sample. Aspiration of the vitreous also may provide material for cytologic examination. The presence of large numbers of eosinophilic indicates a parasitic infection (Figure 5.10). Diagnosis of toxocariasis also may be confirmed by skin testing, and the antigen of toxocara produces an immediate wheal and flare reaction in sensitized individuals.

Treatment

Vitrectomy may be indicated to prevent tractional retinal detachment. The treatment of ocular toxocariasis includes the use of systemic steroids, specifically when the larva dies in the ocular tissues, provoking intense inflammatory reactions. Surgical intervention may be indicated in certain cases. Steroid therapy and photocoagulation of suitable lesions may be considered.

Table 5.3. Visceral and Ocular Larva Migrans

	Visceral Larva Migrans	Ocular Larva Migrans
Mean age of onset	2 years	8 years
Fever	(+)	(−)
Abdominal symptoms (pain, nausea, diarrhea)	(+)	(−)
Nonspecific pulmonary disease	(+)	(−)
Hepatosplenomegaly	(+)	(−)
Eosinophilia	(+)	(−)
Hypergammaglobulinemia	(+)	(−)
Se anti-*Toxocara* antibodies	(+)	(±)
Aqueous anti-*Toxocara* antibodies	(+)	(+)
Ocular findings (uveitis)	(−)	(+)

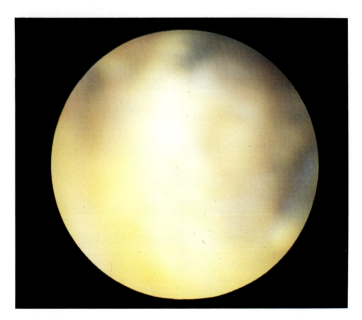

Figure 5.8. Posterior granuloma in a patient with ocular toxocariasis.

Cysticercosis

The larval forms of several species of *Tinea solium* may reach the eye by hematogenous route after the eggs of the worm are ingested by the patient. The eggs of the parasite may reach the stomach by reverse peristalsis. On digestion of the egg walls by gastric enzymes, the larval form of the parasite may migrate throughout the body, including the eye. Cysticerci are the larval forms of the *Tinea solium.* Humans are the natural definitive host. The cys-

ticercus is the larva, which has antigenic fluid in its bladder; on reaching the eye, it may be observed in the vitreous or anterior chamber or the retina (Figure 5.11). When the bladder releases antigenic fluid, it causes considerable inflammation within the eye.

Clinical Findings

Clinical manifestations vary according to location and number of cysts. The location of cysticerci producing disease fall into three anatomic sites: eye,

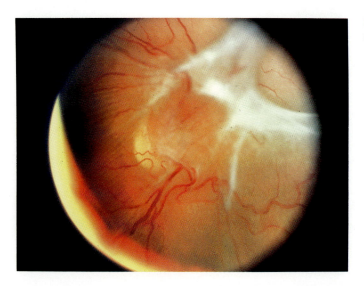

Figure 5.9. Healed ocular toxocariasis with extensive retinal fibrosis.

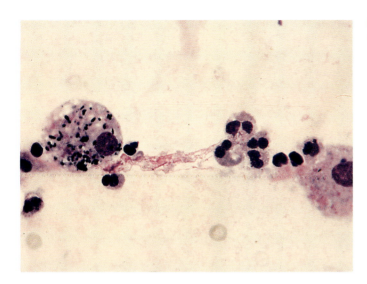

Figure 5.10. Subretinal fluid in a patient with toxocariasis, showing eosinophils.

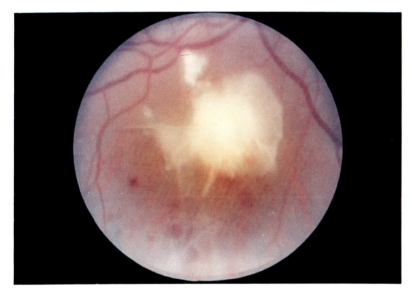

Figure 5.11. Ocular cysticercosis in a 33-year-old man.

brain, and spinal cord and meninges. Loss of vision may be the presenting complaint. Larvae may be in the vitreous, retina, or anterior chamber. Complications include severe intraocular inflammation after death of larva and release of its contents. Iridocyclitis, choroiditis, retinal atrophy, and detachment may occur.

Laboratory Diagnosis

Vitreous specimens may show eosinophils. The diagnosis of cysticercosis is mostly clinical, but ELISA kits and indirect hemagglutination test (IHA) are available for the diagnosis of cestodes in-

festations. Antibodies may be found in the cerebrospinal fluid and serum.

Treatment

Treatment of intraocular cysticercus consists of surgical removal of cysticercus and systemic steroids, and paraziquantel 50 mg/kg/d for 2 weeks.

Diffuse Unilateral Neuroretinitis

This disease is known to be produced by movement of a larva that may be associated with widespread atrophic changes in the retinal pigment epithelium and may eventuate in severe optic atrophy.[17-23] Several larvae of parasites may lead to this entity. The predominant clinical finding includes focal areas of retinitis vasculitis with retinal hemorrhages, retinal tracks, and subretinal fibrosis. Visual loss is secondary to helminth-induced inflammation of the retina, blood vessels, and optic nerve head. The release of parasitic antigens induces local inflammation within the retina and vitreous cavity.

Gass and co-workers[19] were successful in identifying viable intraretinal nematode larvae in two patients with diffuse unilateral subacute neuroretinitis. Gass established that diffuse unilateral subacute neuroretinitis is a form of ocular larva migrans.[19-21] The disease, however, may be caused by other helminth besides nematodes. McDonald and associates[17] reported two cases of intraocular infection with mesocercariae of a trematode known as *Alaria.* The patients were 35- and 38-year-old Asian males living in San Francisco, California. In both patients pigmentary tracks were noted in the retina with areas of active or healed retinitis. The probable source of infection was presumed to be the ingestion of undercooked frogs legs containing *Alaria.* The most common cause of diffuse unilateral subacute neuroretinitis is the larvae of certain nematodes such as *Toxocara canis* of dogs and *Baylisascaris procyonis* of raccoons.[18]

Ankylostoma caninum, the dog hookworm, has been suggested as a cause of diffuse unilateral subacute neuroretinitis. The death of a larva within the ocular structures induces a fulminant uveitis.[24] This requires systemic therapy with corticosteriods. Laser photocoagulation is effective for subretinal or intraretinal worms.[20] Vitrectomy to remove intravitreal and subretinal worms has also been reported as an effective treatment. Gass and associates[25] have successfully treated cases of diffuse unilateral subacute neuroretinitis with oral thiabendazole. Ivermectin may also be used in the treatment of nematodal infection but has not been tried in patients with diffuse unilateral subacute neuroretinitis. Agents that are effective against nematodes such as ivermectin, thiabendazole, and diethylcarbamazine, are not effective in the treatment of trematodes such as *Alaria.* Praziquantel and albendazole may be used in the therapy of trematodol infections. The use of oral antiparasitic agents in diffuse unilateral subacute neuroretinitis may be of limited value in cases with dead larvae or in cases where the larva is in the vitreous. Oral prednisone 1 to 2 mg/kg/d may be helpful in decreasing the intraocular inflammation.

References

1. Masur H, Jones TC, Lempert JA, Cherubini TD: Outbreak of toxoplasmosis in a family and documentation of acquired retinochoroiditis. Am J Med 1978;64:396–402.
2. Michelson JB, Shields JA, McDonald PR, et al.: Retinitis secondary to acquired systemic toxoplasmosis with isolation of the parasite. Am J Ophthalmol 1978;86:548–552.
3. Silveira C, Belfort R Jr, Burnier M Jr, et al.: Acquired toxoplasmic infection as the cause of toxoplasmic retinochoroiditis in families. Am J Ophthalmol 1988;106(3):362–364.
4. Teutsch SM, Juranek DD, Sulzer A, et al.: Epidemic toxoplasmosis associated with infected cats. N Engl J Med 1979;300:695–699.
5. Ryning FW, McCleod R, Maddox JC, et al.: Probable transmission of *Toxoplasma gondii* by organ transplantation. Ann Intern Med 1979;90:47–49.
6. Brezin AP, Egwuagu CE, Burnier M Jr., et al.: Identification of *Toxoplasma gondii* in paraffin-embedded sections by the polymerase chain reaction. Am J Ophthalmol 1990;110:599–604.
7. Tabbara KF, O'Connor GR: Treatment of ocular toxoplasmosis with clindamycin and sulfadiazine. Ophthalmology 1980;87:129.
8. Tate GW, Martin RG: Clindamycin in the treatment of human ocular toxoplasmosis. Can J Ophthalmol 1977;12:188.
9. Tabbara KF, O'Connor GR: Ocular tissue absorption of clindamycin phosphate. Arch Ophthalmol 1975;93:1180–1185.
10. Tabbara KF, Dy-Liacco J, Nozik RA, et al.: Clindamycin in chronic toxoplasmosis: Effect of periocular injections on recoverability of organisms from healed lesions in the rabbit eye. Arch Ophthalmol 1979;97:542–544.
11. Rollins DF, Tabbara KF, Ghosheh R, Nozik RA: Minocycline in experimental ocular toxoplasmosis in the rabbit. Am J Ophthalmol 1982;93:361–365.
12. Engstrom RE, Holland GN, Nussenblatt RB, Jabs DA: Current practices in the management of ocular toxoplasmosis. Am J Ophthalmol 1991;111:601.
13. O'Connor GR, Frenkel JK: Dangers of steroid treatment in toxoplasmosis. Arch Ophthalmol 1976;94:213.
14. Guerina NG, Hsu H-W, Meissner C, et al.: Neonatal serologic screening and early treatment for congenital *Toxoplasma gondii* infection. N Engl J Med 1994;330:1858–1863.
15. Remington JS, Desmonts G: Toxoplasmosis. In Remington JS, Klein JO, eds. Infectious Diseases of the Fe-

tus and Newborn Infant, 3rd ed. Philadelphia: W.B. Saunders, 1990;89–195.

16. Buissonniere RF, De Boissieu D, Tell G, et al.: Uveomeningitis revealing a West African trypanosomiasis in a 12 year-old girl. Arch Fr Pediatr 1989;46(7):517–519.

17. McDonald HR, Kazacos KR, Schatz H, Johnson RN: Two cases of intraocular infection with *Alaria* mesocercaria (Trematoda). Am J Ophthalmol 1994;117:447–455.

18. Kazacos KR: Visceral and ocular larva migrans. Semin Vet Med Surg (Small Anim) 1991;6:227.

19. Gass JD, Gilbert WR, Jr., Guerry RK, Scelfo R: Diffuse unilateral subacute neuroretinitis. Ophthalmology 1978; 85:521.

20. Gass JD, Braunstein RA: Further observations concerning the diffuse unilateral subacute neuroretinitis syndrome. Arch Ophthalmol 1983;101:1689.

21. Gass JD: Stereoscopic Atlas of Macular Diseases. Diagnosis and Treatment, 3rd ed., Vol 2. St. Louis: CV Mosby 1987, pp. 470–475.

22. Kasacos KR, Raymond LA, Kazacos EA, Vestre WA: The raccoon oscarid. A probable cause of human ocular larva migrans. Ophthalmology 1985;92:1735.

23. Goldberg MA, Kazocos KR, Boyce WM, et al.: Diffuse unilateral subacute neuroretinitis in California. Ophthalmology 1993;100:1695.

24. Byers B, Kimura SJ: Uveitis after death of a larva in the vitreous cavity. Am J Ophthalmol 1974;77:63.

25. Gass JD, Callanan D, Bowman CB: Oral therapy in diffuse unilateral subacute neuroretinitis. Arch Ophthalmol 1992;110:675.

Onchocerciasis

Onchocerciasis is a parasitic disease caused by the filarial worm *Onchocerca volvulus* and is a major cause of world blindness. Approximately one million people in the world suffer a significant visual loss from onchocerciasis, and up to 85.5 million live in the endemic areas and are therefore exposed to the risk of this disease.[1] The disease is widely endemic in tropical Africa and in Yemen and in isolated foci in Central and South America. The transmission of *O. volvulus* requires the intervention of a vector, the biting black fly of the genus Simulium, which breeds along fast-moving streams. Different species can carry the disease, but the most important species is *Simulium damnosum.* The dependence of the vector on water courses accounts for the focal distribution of communities suffering from onchocerciasis and explains why the disease is commonly called "river-blindness." It is the ocular lesions of onchocerciasis that cause the true disablement and that, in the worst affected areas, account for the so-

cioeconomic disaster of desertion and depopulation of the fertile land near the rivers. Furthermore, the mortality rate among adult blind persons in the affected villages is three to four times as high as among sighted persons in the same age group.[2]

The worms may host in human body for up to 20 years, and during that time the female worm produces millions of microfilariae, which are found in the highest concentrations in the skin and the eyes of the host. Adult worms coil together in the fibrous nodules (onchocercomas), which lie either subcutaneously or deep in the tissues. Heavily infected people often tolerate the adult worms and the living microfilariae surprisingly well. Only a very small proportion of the microfilariae are ingested by a feeding Simulium vector; the overwhelming majority of the microfilariae die in the tissues, causing inflammation and scars, which result in blindness and other characteristic symptoms.

Onchocerciasis is characterized by subcutaneous nodules, ocular, lymphatic, and dermal lesions. Major changes in ocular onchocerciasis can occur in almost all ocular tissues, but blindness usually results from sclerosing keratitis, chorioretinal lesions, and optic atrophy or secondary glaucoma. The posterior segment involvement indicates an advanced disease and forms a poor prognostic sign.[3]

Clinical Manifestations

Ocular involvement in onchocerciasis includes the presence of either living or dead microfilariae in the eye, resulting in corneal disease (punctate keratitis, snowflake opacities, sclerosing keratitis), iridocyclitis (frequently associated with secondary cataract and glaucoma), chorioretinal lesions, optic neuritis, and disc atrophy. There is a great difference between the presence of living microfilariae and the inflammatory reaction, which they apparently produce when they die. It is quite common to see an eye that contains many microfilariae, but shows very little evidence of inflammation. The pathologic changes develop slowly; even in the areas that are heavily infested with *Onchocerca volvulus,* it usually takes many years to cause severe visual loss.

A geographical classification of the clinical disease into the savanna form and the rain forest form is widely used: the savanna form is characterized by more predominant sclerosing keratitis and iritis and carries a worse visual prognosis, whereas the prevalence of chorioretinitis was similar in both areas.[4,5] The considerable variation in the severity of the disease exists, probably attributable to the pathogenicity of the various vector–parasite complexes.

Scleritis, episcleritis, and limbal microabscess are usually observed after treatment with microfilaricides, but also can be found in untreated patients. Corneal snowflake opacities are transient and usually disappear after several weeks or after treatment. The irreversible form of the corneal disease is called sclerosing keratitis. In the beginning there is an opacification of the cornea in the nasal and temporal part of the interpalpebral fissure, which later extends inferiority in a semilunar form, and finally moves upwards and covers the pupillary aperture, which results in the loss of visual acuity. A high microfilarial load of the anterior chamber is an important risk factor for blindness and is strongly associated with the occurrence of severe posterior segment changes.[6] The parasites sometimes concentrated in the lower angle of the anterior chamber, causing an inflammation with a secondary "onchopupil" (pear-shaped pupillary aperture with apex downwards, usually associated with secondary cataract and a bad reaction to light). The vitreal microfilariae and the netlike vitreal filaments have been documented.[7]

The exact incidence of chorioretinal lesions in onchocerciasis is not known; in the field situation these lesions are not systematically assessed and can be masked by media opacities (sclerosing keratitis, cataract). In an isolated savanna onchocerciasis focus in Ghana, an overall incidence of chorioretinal changes was seen in 12% of the onchocerciasis patients[8]; in another series of onchocerciasis patients with ocular involvement from a hyperendemic area in Sierra Leone, all of whom had consulted the eye hospital with visual complaints, 48% had chorioretinal alterations typical of onchocerciasis.[3] The posterior segment/lesions occur in severely infected patients and increase sharply after the age of 30 years.[9]

Evaluation of posterior segment changes attributable to onchocerciasis is not consistent. In the past, little attention was directed toward the importance of chorioretinal alterations and optic disc atrophy, because blinding conditions in patients with onchocerciasis. Bird and co-workers reported that optic nerve disease, alone or in combination with chorioretinal lesions, was responsible for blindness in 88% of patients with posterior pole involvement.[5]

Fundus changes are usually bilateral, but not always symmetrical. In a series of 244 patients with posterior pole involvement, three grades of retinal involvement could be recognized.[5] The chorioretinal lesions usually start temporal to the macula and consist of small punctate epithelial dots and occasional cotton-wool spots (grade 1, Figure 5.12). Pigment mottling may progress to focal atrophy of pigment epithelium and choroidal capillaries (Grade 2, Figure 5.13). Characteristic are the sharply demarcated borders of atrophic and normal retinal tissue. Focal areas of chorioretinal atrophy usually occur in a (incomplete) ring formation, which encircles the macula, frequently sparing the isolated remnants of the normal retinal tissue. This distribution was attributed to the presumed passage of the microfilariae into the eye through the scleral canals along the entry of short ciliary arteries. Later in the disease process, the confluent areas of chorioretinal atrophy almost affect the whole of retina and choroid (Grade 3, Figure 5.14). and subretinal fibrosis may be visible. Pigment clumping is characteristic for these advanced atrophic lesions and the aspect may resemble tapetoretinal dystrophy. The whitish infiltrates can sometimes be seen, usually located on the border or within an atrophic area and may show excessive leakage on fluorescein angiography. The distinction between active retinal inflammation and secondary fibrosis is very difficult because the vitreous is clear in most cases. Sheathing of the big retinal vessels may be present, either isolated or in combination with chorioretinal or optic disc lesions.

Optic nerve involvement includes active neuritis with a swelling of the optic disc, but more frequently partial or total atrophy is encountered. Sometimes, evidence of previous inflammation is apparent (gliosis, pigmentations around the disc, and sheathing of the vessels).[10–16] Optic atrophy is probably an important cause of visual loss. This visual loss may follow any pattern, but most commonly presents with a constriction of the visual fields and night blindness. In 93% (137/148) of the patients with optic disc atrophy, associated chorioretinal lesions were present; however, most of these changes were mild, so that it was considered unlikely that the optic atrophy was consecutive to chorioretinal disease.[5] Ophthalmologic examination antibodies against a human retinal extract and bovine S-antigen in onchocerciasis patients.[17] Chan and

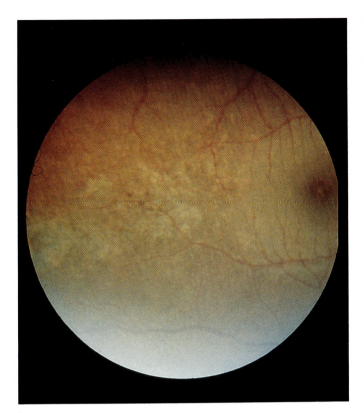

A

Figure 5.12. Chorioretinal lesions in onchocerciasis, grade 1. **A** and **B:** Irregular atrophy of pigment epithelium temporal to the macula showing mottled appearance.

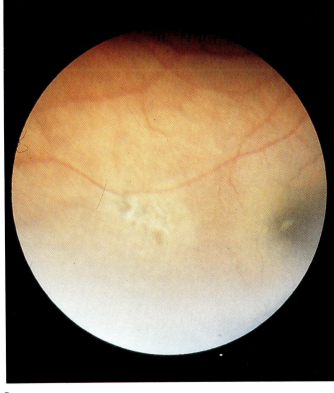

B

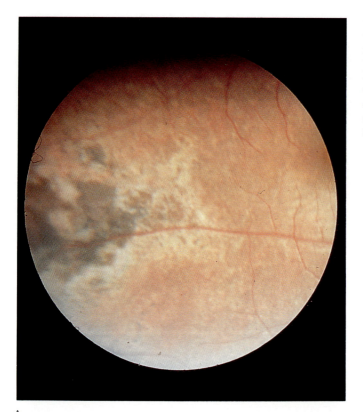

Figure 5.13. Chorioretinal lesions in onchocerciasis, grade 2. **A.** Focal atrophy of pigment epithelium and choriocapillaris as well as secondary hyperpigmentations. **B.** More extended atrophy of pigment epithelium and choriocapillaris; large choroidal vessels are visible. Noteworthy are the sharply demarcated borders of atrophic area and concurrent optic disc atrophy.

A

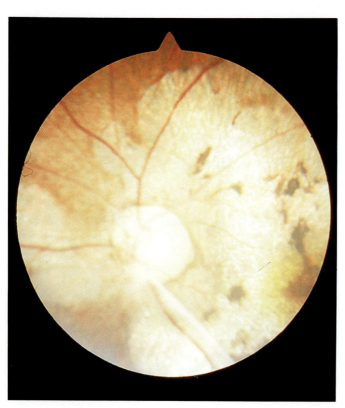

B

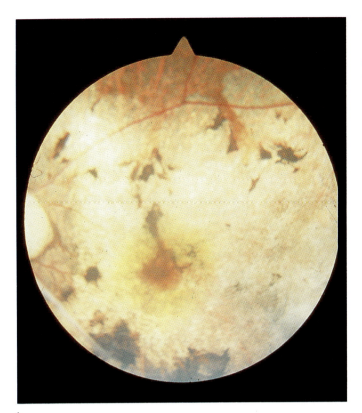

Figure 5.14. Chorioretinal lesions in onchocerciasis, grade 3. **A.** and **B.:** Widespread atrophy of choroid and retina with pigment clumping. A remnant of "normal" retinal tissue is left around the fovea.

A

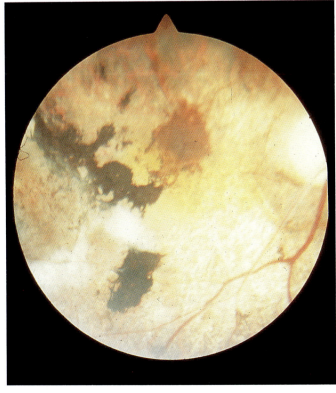

B

co-workers found antibodies against inner retina in 10 of 12 patients with onchocerciasis and in 3 of 9 controls.[18] Van der Lelij and co-workers observed high levels of antiretinal antibodies (human S-antigen and human interphotoreceptor retinoid-binding protein, IRBP) in onchocerciasis patients without ocular involvement and endemic controls as well as in patients with other filarial infections, which do not cause an ocular disease.[19] Cell-mediated immune responses to the human retinal S-antigen, IRBP, and crude retinal extract did not differ in patients with or without onchocercal retinopathy or in endemic controls.[20] Therefore it seems unlikely that a humoral or cell-mediated immunity against retinal antigens plays an important role in the pathogenesis of the atrophic retinal lesions.

Clinical findings suggest that retinal alterations can be attributed directly to the microfilariae or their toxins, because the progression of retinal changes after treatment with ivermectin occurred only in patients with an evidence of active onchocerciasis at that time. Also the adverse ocular reactions to microfilaricidal drugs support this hypothesis, as well as the histologic evidence of microfilariae in the retina and choroid. An experimental model of onchocercal retinal lesions in the cynomolgus monkey has indicated that active infiltration of the retina by microfilariae may lead to a progressive widespread chorioretinal damage.[21] In clinical terms, it is likely that other factors such as prenatal sensitization, duration of the infection and its parasital load, previous treatments, and the patient's age are also important.

Laboratory Findings

The most reliable proof of onchocerciasis remains the detection of the parasite. This is usually performed by the so-called skin-snip test, in which a small fragment of skin is put in saline or a tissue culture medium and, after a few minutes, the microfilariae may be seen moving actively by using a low-power microscope.[22] The assessment of the microfilarial load of the skin is an important factor, predicting the level of parasites in the eye and is strongly correlated with the frequency of side effects after therapy.[23–25] In the field situation a simple variant of the test has to be sufficient, whereas in more fortunate circumstances or for research purposes the quantification of the number of microfilariae per mg skin is recommended. A simple razor blade or a corneal punch is used for the skin biopsy. The outer canthus, which has been reported as the best site for the skin biopsy, is painful and often leaves a permanent scar. Therefore skin biopsies are more frequently performed above an iliac crest or a shoulder.

The provocative Mazzotti test assesses the concentration of microfilariae by the patient's reaction to 50 mg diethylcarbamazine. This dose kills the microfilariae and produces a reaction in the patient consisting of itching, which may progress to skin edema, erythema, and papular eruption. More severe cases are accompanied by fever, malaise, joint pain, and lymphadenopathy. The test was widely used in persons with a negative skin-snip test result or whenever the skin-snip could not be performed. However, the Mazzotti reaction can be quite severe in the heavily infected patients.

A reliable immunodiagnostic test is not yet available. An accurate and rapid diagnosis, especially in the early stages of the infection, is becoming increasingly urgent for the control of onchocerciasis. The early detection of (re)infection in the parasite-free areas obtained by the vector or other control programs is especially important. Extensive research is being done using techniques such as monoclonal antibodies, antigen capture assays, recombinant peptides, and polymerase chain reaction (PCR). The mainstay for the diagnosis of onchocerciasis remains the detection of the parasite either in the skin or in the eye, however.

Treatment

A discussion of onchocerciasis treatment should be separated into that of infected individuals under hospital supervision and that applied for control of the disease within the community.

Onchocerciasis control programs

The possibilities for onchocerciasis control are limited. Until recently, chemotherapy was not an option, because the existing drugs for the treatment of onchocerciasis were unsatisfactory, associated with severe side effects, and were therefore unsuitable for a large-scale treatment. The only alternative was larviciding of the vector's breeding sites over an extensive area and during a long period. This was the approach chosen for the onchocerciasis control program (OCP) in West Africa, which operates under the auspices of the World Health Organization. Despite the many problems the OCP had to overcome, including reinvasion by long-distance migration of the infective vectors from the breeding sites outside the OCP areas, the disease control within the OCP area has been effective. The problem related to the OCP vector control is of enormous geographical and time extent, which is associated with extremely high costs. The reinfection from outside areas, the resistance to multiple insecticides, and obviously the eventual impact of insecticides on the environment are the additional risks.

Ivermectin, a new agent in the field of onchocerciasis, has just become available. An annual dose of ivermectin was reported to be effective in interrupting transmission of *Onchocerca volvulus* for an extended period.[26,27] The adverse reactions associated with initial ivermectin dose were common and occurred mostly within 48 hours after treatment.[23,24] The side effects were usually mild and could be managed successfully. The frequency and severity of adverse reactions were found to be related to the degree of parasite infestation of the patient[23,24] and decreased after repeated treatments.[28] Annual mass chemotherapy with ivermectin in addition to the original vector control strategy is planned for the future.

Treatment of Ocular Onchocerciasis.

Most pathologic changes in the eye area are irreversible, and the basic aim of treatment is to stop the disease and prevent any further loss of sight. The traditional treatment for onchocerciasis consisted of a course of diethylcarbamazine (DEC) and suramin. However, this therapy was associated with serious, even fatal adverse reactions and aggravation of ocular lesions, including irreversible posterior segment changes.[29–36]

Since its registration for use in human onchocerciasis in 1988, ivermectin is the treatment of choice for ocular onchocerciasis. All published reports comparing ivermectin with diethylcarbamazine therapy agree that ivermectin is a better tolerated, safer, and more effective agent.[37–41] After a single oral dose of ivermectin (150 μg/kg) given to adult patients, the microfilarial densities in the skin and in the eyes remained low for up to 1 year, probably because of the combination of a microfilaricidal ef-

fect and the inhibition of the release of microfilaria from the adult worm uterus.[37,42,43]

These studies included mostly patients with a mild ocular disease; there is no consensus yet concerning the best therapy for individual patients, especially those with severe ocular onchocerciasis from a hyperendemic area, treated with a 6-monthly ivermectin dose, one-third of the patients had persistent active ocular disease (including progressive chorioretinal lesions) in a follow-up period of 6 and 12 months.[3] This indicates that even a 6-monthly dose of ivermectin is not sufficient to stop the progression of ocular disease in severely infected patients. Until now, higher-dosage regimens could not be associated with better therapeutic results.[44–46] The persistence of active ocular onchocerciasis despite treatment was related to the pretreatment severity of ocular disease. Assessment of the ocular status was a valuable guide to therapy and should be attempted by all clinicians.

The reported ocular side effects of ivermectin therapy include a short-term mobilization of microfilariae into the anterior chamber, mild anterior uveitis, and posterior segment changes consisting of transient or minor pigment epithelial alterations and temporarily increased disc hyperfluorescence.[39,40,44,45] New infiltrates within the already damaged retinal areas occurred after ivermectin therapy in 3 of 32 patients with chorioretinal lesions.[23] The patients with ocular onchocerciasis have more frequent and more serious adverse reactions after ivermectin treatment, because these side effects are closely related to the degree of parasitic infestation.

Until now, there is no effective and acceptable therapeutical agent against the adult worm. The excision of onchocercal nodules was reported not to be beneficial.

Conclusion

Optic disc atrophy and chorioretinal lesions are frequently the cause of visual handicap in onchocerciasis. The pathogenesis of chorioretinal lesions is not known, but probably can be attributed to the severe reaction that occurs after death of microfilariae in the posterior segment. Posterior segment involvement indicates an advanced disease and carries a bad ocular prognosis. The new era of chemotherapy in onchocerciasis treatment has started with the use of ivermectin, a highly effective drug and in community trials rarely associated with serious side effects.

Onchocerciasis occurs mainly in isolated areas with little or no health care facilities. In most countries affected by onchocerciasis, there is also a high incidence of various other diseases caused by poor hygiene and poor nutrition. The medical profession is concerned with treating and preventing disease, and yet most doctors have chosen to work in those areas where most people are healthy.

The attempted goal of OCP, "to control onchocerciasis as a disease of public health and socio-economic importance and to ensure that there will be no recrudescence of the disease thereafter," will be very difficult to achieve because there is apparently little awareness of this problem, although it is one of the most important but avoidable causes of visual handicap worldwide.

References

1. WHO Expert Committee on Onchocerciasis, Third Report. Technical Report Series 752. World Health Organization, Geneva, 1987:8–21.
2. Prost A, Vaugelade J: La surmortalite' des aveugles en zone de savane ouest-africaine. Bull WHO 1981;59: 773–776.
3. Rothova MA, Van der Lelij A, Stilma JS, et al.: Ocular involvement in onchocerciasis after repeated treatment with ivermectin. Am J Ophthalmol 1990;110:6–16.
4. Andreson J, Fuglsang H, Hamilton PJS, Marshall TF de C: Studies on onchocerciasis in the United Cameroon Republic II. Comparison of populations in rain forest and Sudan savanna. Trans R Soc Trop Med Hyg 1974; 68:209–222.
5. Bird AC, Anderson J, Fuglsang H: Morphology of posterior segment lesions of the eye in patients with onchocerciasis. Br J Ophthalmol 1976;60:2–20.
6. Thylefors B, Brinkmann UK: The microfilarial load in the anterior segment of the eye: A parameter of intensity of onchocerciasis. Bull WHO 1977;55:731–737.
7. Reyna O, Flores Z, Nowell de Arevalo AM, et al.: Ultrasound detection of changes in the vitreous humor of onchocerciasis patients from Guatemala. Trans R Soc Trop Med Hyg 1988;82:606.
8. Dadzie KY, Remme J, Alley ES, de Sole, G: Changes in ocular onchocerciasis four and twelve months after community-based treatment with ivermectin in a holo-endemic onchocerciasis focus. Trans R Soc Trop Med Hyg 1990;84:103–108.
9. Berghout E: Onchocerciasis and optic atrophy in the savannah area of Ghana. Tropical and Geographical Medicine 1987;39:323–329.
10. Murphy RP, Taylor H, Greene BM: Chorioretinal damage in onchocerciasis. Am J Ophthalmol 1984;98: 519–521.
11. Neumann E, Gunders AE. Pathogenesis of the posterior segment lesion of ocular onchocerciasis. Am J Ophthalmol 1973;75:82–89.
12. Garner A, Duke BOL: Fundus lesions in the rabbit eye following inoculation of Onchocerca volvulus microfilariae into the posterior segment. Tropenmed Parasit 1976;27:19–29.
13. Ridley H: Ocular onchocerciasis, including an investigation in the Gold Coast. Br J Ophthalmol 1945; (Suppl.):10.
13a. Lopez JS, de Smet MD, Masur H, et al.: Orally administered 566C 80 for treatment of ocular toxoplasmosis in a patient with the acquired immunodeficiency syndrome. Am J Ophthalmol 1992;113:331–333.
14. Rodger FC, The pathogenesis and pathology of ocular onchocerciasis. Part III. The posterior segment lesion. Am J Ophthalmol 1960;49:127–135.
15. Rockey JH, Donnelly JJ, Stromberg BE, Soulsby EJL: Immunopathology of toxocara canis and Ascaris suum infections of the eye; the role of the eosinophil. Invest Ophthalmol Vis Sci 1979;18:1172–1184.
16. O'Day J, Mackenzie CD: Ocular onchocerciasis: Diagnosis and current clinical approaches. Tropical Doctor 1985;15:87–94.
17. Vingtain P, Thillaye B, Karpouzas I, Faure JP: Longitudinal study of microfilarial infestation and humoral immune response to filarial and retinal antigens in onchocerciasis patients treated with ivermectin. Ophthalmic Res 1988;20:61–98.
18. Chan CC, Nussenblatt RB, Kim MK, et al.: Immunopathology of ocular onchocerciasis. 2. Anti-retinal autoantibodies in serum and ocular fluids. Ophthalmology 1987;94:439–443.
19. Van der Lelij A, Doekes G, Hwan BS, et al.: Humoral autoimmune response against S-antigen and IRBP in ocular onchocerciasis. Invest Ophthalmol Vis Sci 1990;31: 180–186.
20. Van der Lelij A, Rothova A, Stilma JS, et al.: Cell-mediated immunity against human retinal extract, S-antigen and interphotoreceptor retinoid binding protein in onchocercal chorioretinopathy. Invest Ophthalmol Vis Sci 1990;31:2031–2036.
21. Semba RD, Donnelly JJ, Rockey JH, et al.: Experimental ocular onchocerciasis in Cynomolgus Monkeys. II. Chorioretinitis elicited by intravitreal Onchocerca lienalis microfilariae. Invest Ophthalmol Vis Sci 1988;29: 1642–1651.
22. Sandford-Smith J: Eye diseases in hot climates. Bristol: John Wright and Sons Ltd. 1986:180.
23. Rothova A, Van der Lelij A, Stilma JS, et al.: Side effects of ivermectin in treatment of onchocerciasis. Lancet 1989;1:1439–1441.
24. De Sole G, Awadzi K, Remme J, et al.: A community trial of ivermectin in the onchocerciasis focus of

Asubende, Ghana. II. Adverse reactions. Trop Med Parasit 1989;40:375–382.

25. Anderson J, Fuglsang H, Hamilton PJS, Marshall TF de C: The prognostic value of head nodules and microfilariae in the skin in relation to ocular onchocerciasis. Tropenmed Parasit 1975;26:191–195.

26. Cupp EW, Bernardo MJ, Kiszewski AE, et al.: The effects of ivermectin on transmission of Onchocerca volvulus. Science 1986;231:740.

27. Albiez EJ, Newland HS, White AT, et al.: Chemotherapy of onchocerciasis with high doses of diethylcarbamazine or a single dose of ivermectin: Microfilaria levels and side-effects. Trop Med Parasitol 1988;39:19.

28. De Sole G, Dadzie KY, Giese J, Remme J. Lack of adverse reactions in ivermectin treatment of onchocerciasis. Lancet 1990;i:1106–1107.

29. Oomen AP. Fatalities after treatment of onchocerciasis with diethylcarbamazine. Trans R Soc Trop Med Hyg 1969;63:548.

30. Fuglsang H, Anderson J: Collapse during treatment of onchocerciasis with diethylcarbamazine. Trans R Soc Trop Med Hyg 1974;68:72–73.

31. Anderson J, Fuglsang H: Effects of Diethylcarbamazine on ocular onchocerciasis. Tropenmed Parasit 1976;27:263–278.

32. Bryceson ADM, Warrell DA, Pope HM: Dangerous reactions to treatment of onchocerciasis with diethylcarbamazine. Br Med J 1977;1:742–744.

33. Thylefors B, Rolland A: The risk of optic atrophy following suramin treatment of ocular onchocerciasis. Bull WHO 1979;3:479–480.

34. Bird AC, El Sheikh H, Anderson J, Fuglsang H: Changes in visual function and in the posterior segment of the eye during treatment of onchocerciasis with diethylcarbamazine citrate. Br J Ophthalmol 1980;64:191–200.

35. Taylor HR, Greene BM: Ocular changes with oral and transepidermal diethylcarbamazine therapy of onchocerciasis. Br J Ophthalmol 1981;65:494–502.

36. Greene BM, Taylor HR, Brown EJ, et al.: Ocular and systemic complications of diethylcarbamazine therapy for onchocerciasis: Association with circulating immune complexes. J Infect Dis 1983;147:890–897.

37. Lariviere M, Vingtain P, Aziz MA, et al.: Double-blind study of ivermectin and diethylcarbamazine in African onchocerciasis patients with ocular involvement. Lancet 1985;ii:174–177.

38. Greene BM, Taylor HR, Cupp EW, et al.: Comparison of ivermectin and diethylcarbamazine in the treatment of onchocerciasis. N Engl J Med 1985;313:133–138.

39. Taylor HR, Murphy RP, Newland HS, et al.: Treatment of onchocerciasis: The ocular effects of ivermectin and diethylcarbamazine. Arch Ophthalmol 1986;104:863–870.

40. Dadzie KY, Bird AC, Awadzi K, et al.: Ocular findings in a double-blind study of ivermectin versus diethylcarbamazine versus placebo in the treatment of onchocerciasis. Br J Ophthalmol 1987;71:78–85.

41. Albiez EJ, Newland HS, White AT, et al.: Chemotherapy of onchocerciasis with high doses of diethylcarbamazine or a single dose of ivermectin: microfilaria levels and side effects. Trop Med Parasit 1988;39:19–24.

42. Soboslay PT, Newland HS, White AT, et al.: Ivermectin effect on microfilariae of Onchocerca volvulus after a single oral dose in humans. Trop Med Parasit 1987;38:8–10.

43. Albiez EJ, Walter G, Kaiser A, et al.: Histological examination of onchocercomata after therapy with ivermectin. Trop Med Parasit 1988;39:93–99.

44. Awadzi K, Dadzie KY, Schulz-Key H, et al.: The chemotherapy of onchocerciasis X. Ann Trop Med Parasitol 1985;79:63–78.

45. Dadzie KY, Awadzi K, Bird AC, Schulz-Key H: Ophthalmological results from a placebo controlled comparative 3-dose ivermectin study in the treatment of onchocerciasis. Trop Med Parasit 1989;40:355–360.

46. Taylor HR, Semba RD, Newland HS, et al.: Ivermectin treatment of patients with severe ocular onchocerciasis. Am J Trop Med Hyg 1989;40:494–500.

47. Fuglsang H, Anderson J: Further observations on the relationship between ocular onchocerciasis and the head nodule, and on the possible benefit of nodulectomy. Br J Ophthalmol 1978;62:445–449.

Chapter 6
Fungal Infections

Khalid F. Tabbara

Candidiasis

Candidiasis is a disease that is caused by the fungus *Candida*. Candida infections of the mucous membrane are not uncommon in humans. Invasive candidiasis occurs in patients with immunologic suppression.[1-5] The disease is common among patients with acquired immune deficiency syndrome, patients on hyperalimentation or immunosuppressive agents, patients with malignancy, and patients with indwelling catheters.

Clinical Findings

Intraocular infection with *Candida* species occurs after candidemia. The lesion usually appears in the choriocapillaries or in the superficial retina. The organism is a yeast fungus that grows in tissues as pseudohyphae. These forms extend throughout the tissues and may grow into the vitreous, breaking the barrier of the inner limiting membrane of the retina. The early lesion of intraocular infection presents as a focal area of whitish elevated retinitis. Lesions may appear as multiple foci of retinitis with subjacent choroiditis. The lesion may progress into the vitreous cavity. Multiple small foci may disclose stringy connections and may give the appearance of a string of pearls, which is characteristic of *Candida* infections of the retina (Figure 6.1). Occasionally initial lesions may be misdiagnosed as toxoplasmic retinochoroiditis. The underlying vitreous appears to be clear in the initial stages of the disease, but a few days later shows snowballs in the vitreous.

Each of those snowballs consists of focal infection with *Candida* species. The disease may progress to panophthalmitis if not identified early and treated promptly. Progression of the disease is relentless with eventual organization of the vitreous leading to retinal detachment. Anterior iridocyclitis associated with pain and photophobia as well as secondary glaucoma may occur.

Laboratory Diagnosis

The precipitant test for *Candida* infection detects the presence of circulating precipitating antibodies to the organism. Patients with precipitating antibodies in their sera may be either acutely or chronically infected. False-negative reactions may occur. Immune electrophoresis has been used to increase the diagnostic accuracy of precipitating antibodies. *Candida* antigens may be detected in ocular fluid specimens or in the blood. Increased levels of D-Arabinitol are found in serum and vitreous specimen.[6] The use of skin testing to detect delayed hypersensitivity to *Candida* is of no value because most of the patients show a positive skin test to *Candida* extracts. Failure to find a positive skin test to *Candida* is generally considered to be a pathologic sign that may indicate the presence of suppressed cell-mediated immunity. The disease progresses to panuveitis and endophthalmitis. Vitreous aspirates are recommended (Figure 6.2), and they should be subjected to Giemsa staining, Gram staining, and methanamine-silver-Gomori stain. Vitreous aspirates also should be subjected

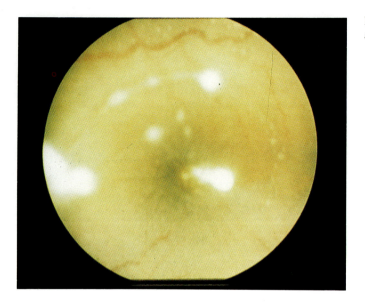

Figure 6.1. Candida retinitis showing focal area of retinitis and string of pearl sign.

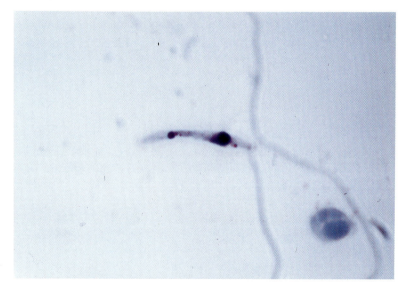

Figure 6.2. Vitreous tap showing pseudohyphae in a patient with candidiasis.

to cultures on appropriate media for the recovery of the organism. Culture of the organism is achieved by placing the specimens on Sabouraud's medium or blood agar. Vitrectomy may be performed immediately after performing a vitreous aspiration.

Treatment

The treatment of *Candida* retinitis and endophthalmitis consists of the systemic administration of amphotericin B. Table 6.1 outlines the regimen rec-

ommended for the use of amphotericin B. In patients with excessive vitreous involvement, a vitrectomy should be performed together with the intraocular injection of 0.5 mg amphotericin B intravitreally. *Candida* retinitis may occur in patients who are drug addicts or immunosuppressed. The cause of immunosuppression should be determined and corrected if possible. Immunosuppressive therapy may be decreased or discontinued whenever possible. Liposomal amphotericin B (AmBisome®) has been made available.[7] Patients with fungal infections may be treated with Liposomal ampho-

Table 6.1. Suggestions on the Use of Amphotericin B*

1. Add 10 mL sterile, preservative-free water to the vial (concentration of drug, 5 mg/mL). (Amphotericin B [Fungizone] is provided in vials containing 50 mg lyophilized drug). This reconstituted concentrate should be used as soon as possible after preparation. It may be kept up to 1 week under refrigeration and 48 hours at room temperature.
2. The dose to be delivered is diluted in the appropriate amount of D5W (see 3 below). This second dilution must be used immediately because deterioration occurs with storage.
3. Dosage schedule
   Day 1: Begin with 1 mg amphotericin B in 500 mL D5W.
   Day 2: 5 mg amphotericin B in 500 mL D5W over 4 to 6 hours.
   Day 3: 10 mg amphotericin B in 500 mL D5W over 4 to 6 hours.
   Day 4: 15 mg amphotericin in 500 mL D5W over 4 to 6 hours.
   Day 5 and thereafter: Dosage is governed by patient's tolerance of the drug, the effect on renal function, and the clinical picture.
   Generally, begin with 20 mg in 1,000 mL D5W over 4 to 6 hours. The rate of administration is varied with tolerance.
4. Expected complications and their amelioration
   a. Thrombophlebitis: Use veins as distal as possible. Use pediatric scalp vein needles; alternate veins from day to day. Add 5 mg heparin to each bottle of drug.
   b. Fever and chills: Give aspirin and chlorpheniramine as needed and vary dose of amphotericin.
   c. Nausea and vomiting: Give chlorpromazine as needed and vary rate of administration of amphotericin.
   d. Anorexia, myalgias, headache: Administer aspirin.
   e. If b, c, and d persist and threaten to interfere with therapy, may add 5–20 mg/day hydrocortisone sodium succinate (Solu-Cortef, Upjohn, Kalamazoo, MI) to intravenous fluid.
   f. Hypokalemia (progression to paralysis has been reported): Determine potassium level.
   g. Azotemia: Determine blood urea nitrogen (BUN) (withhold drug if BUN is greater than 50).
   h. Anemia: Intravenous mannitol may be used to decrease renal toxicity. Determine packed cell volume.

*Tabbara KF: Ocular candidosis, in Tabbara KF, Hyndiuk RA: Infections of the eye. Boston: Little, Brown, & Co., 1986.

tericin B 2 mg/kg/day IV. The drug has been shown to have less toxicity than amphotericin B.[7]

Fluconazole, an imidazole, has been shown to possess pharmacokinetic properties characterized by low lipid solubility and low affinity for plasma proteins.[8,9] These characteristics allow fluconazole to diffuse into body tissue and fluids including the cerebrospinal fluid, sputum, skin, and vaginal tissue.[9] Savani and associates[10] have shown adequate penetration of fluconazole in the ocular tissues and fluids in experimental *Candida* endophthalmitis. Fluconazole appears to achieve the highest concentrations in the ocular tissues followed by ketoconazole and itraconazole.[10–12] The ocular fluid bioavailability of fluconazole has been determined in patients with endophthalmitis. Fluconazole appeared to penetrate the aqueous and vitreous readily.[11] The drug also penetrates the aqueous humor of uninflamed rabbit eyes.[10]

Fluconazole has been shown to be safe and effective in the treatment of *Candida* and cryptococcus infections of the eye.[13–16] Systemic administration of fluconazole, with or without the concomitant use of intravitreal amphotericin B, has eventuated in symptomatic cure and improved vision in patients with fungal endophthalmitis.[13,14] No serious adverse effects have been associated with fluconazole ther-

apy. It may be given intravenously or orally. Initial therapy for severe *Candida* endophthalmitis may be at a dosage level of 200 mg/day IV. In patients with severe vitreous exudates, vitrectomy and intraocular injection of amphotericin B 5 μg should be considered. Fluconazole may be given orally at a dosage level of 200 to 400 mg. Amphotericin B at 5 μg dose and miconazole at 25 to 40 μg dose are considered safe for intravitreal administration.[17] No clinical or histopathologic abnormalities have been noted following intravitreal injection of 100 μg of fluconazole in the rabbit.[18] Safety in man following intravitreal injections remains to be determined.

Coccidioidomycosis

This type of fungal infection is of concern to individuals living in regions of the United States and the northern section of Mexico. Filipinos and black individuals are characteristically more susceptible to coccidioidomycosis than are other individuals. In most cases the systemic infection is asymptomatic, and in others it may lead to pneumonia. The disease is transmitted by inhalation of the spores of the fungus.

Clinical Diagnosis

Patients with coccidioidomycosis may develop anterior uveitis. The characteristic posterior segment lesion in coccidioidomycosis is multifocal choroiditis. At autopsy, multiple choroidal lesions with minimal extension into the overlying retina may be seen. The optic nerve may be involved.

The lesions are composed of focal granulomata consisting of the spherules of the fungus with concentric layers of lymphocyte cells epithelioid and giant cells. The spherules of coccidioidomycosis appear to have a peculiar antigen that stimulates delayed hypersensitivity reactions.

Laboratory Diagnosis

Only one per thousand patients infected with coccidioidomycosis are symptomatic. Patients with disseminated choroiditis are usually debilitated or severely ill. The disease is often fatal.

Antibodies to the organism can be detected by serum testing. A precipitant test is also available. In the acute phase of disseminated disease blood cultures may show the presence of the fungus.

Treatment

The treatment of coccidioidomycosis is systemic intravenous administration of amphotericin B (see Table 6.1) IV. Amphotericin B 0.5 to 0.8 mg/kg/day is given for a total cumulative dose of 2 to 2.5 g. Alternate therapy consists of fluconazole 400 mg orally per day. Patients with meningitis may need intrathecal administration of amphotericin B.

Histoplasmosis

Histoplasmosis is a disease caused by *Histoplasma capsulatum.* Most patients with systemic histoplasmosis are asymptomatic. The disease is endemic in the midwestern region of the United States (predominantly in the Ohio River Valley) and may occur sporadically.

Clinical Findings

Patients with presumed ocular histoplasmosis are asymptomatic. When the visually important structures are involved, patients may complain of blurring or distortion of vision. New characteristic signs of presumed ocular histoplasmosis syndrome consist of focal infiltration (Figure 6.3) and annular punched-out small atrophic spots in the fundus with variable amounts of fine pigmentation. Patients may have peripapillary scarring and evidence of subretinal neovascularization, particularly in the macular area, giving rise to the hemorrhagic detachment of the macula. Patients with presumed ocular histoplasmosis have no signs of active inflammation. The vitreous is perfectly clear and there is no sign of cells or exudates. The iris and ciliary body show no evidence of inflammatory reactions.

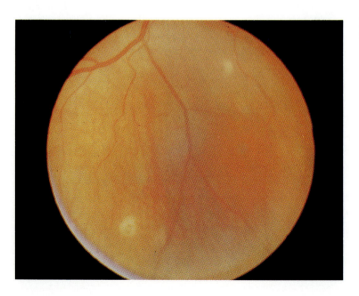

Figure 6.3. *Histoplasma* spot in a patient with presumed ocular histoplasmosis.

Lesions in the fundus are sharply demarcated, appearing completely healed.

Patients who develop atrophic nummular choroidal scars (histo spots) in the posterior pole are at a high risk of developing choroidal neovascularization.[19] Choroidal neovascularization secondary to presumed ocular histoplasmosis occurs adjacent to an atrophic scar.[20–23] It is estimated that out of 70 million people who live in histoplasmosis endemic areas of the United States, 2 million may have histo spots.[24] The risk of blindness and visual impairment among adults 30 years of age or older who have peripheral histo spots only is higher than among control individuals from the same community.[19] In patients with a disciform lesion typical of ocular histoplasmosis in one eye are at risk of developing a disciform lesion in the other eye during a 15-year period.[19] Shields and associates reported a 66-year-old woman who developed an adenocarcinoma of the retinal pigment epithelium arising from a juxtapapillary histoplasmosis scar.[25] The development of a neoplasm from a histoplasma infected ocular structure may be related to a reactive proliferation of the retinal pigment epithelium.

Laboratory Diagnosis

Fluorescein angiography may show window defects in the retinal pigment epithelium showing fluorescence of the underlying choroid. They also may show blockage of the fluorescein associated with choroidal infiltration at the site of the histoplasma fundus spot. Neovascular tufts in the subretinal area may be outlined by fluorescein angiography. A histoplasmin skin test is available. Histoplasma skin testing appears to be the indicator of immunologic activity to histoplasma capsulatum. It should be kept in mind, however, that 11% of patients presenting to eye clinics suffering from presumed ocular histoplasmosis syndrome have negative skin tests.

Treatment

There is no effective therapeutic modality for the treatment of ocular histoplasmosis syndrome. Some patients may benefit from photocoagulation of the subretinal neovascularization areas. Corticosteroids may be of limited value in patients with focal choroiditis. Subretinal neovascularization of the macular area may be treated with photocoagulation.

The Amsler grid is useful to follow patients with macular involvement. If untreated, approximately 60% of the patients may develop a visual acuity of less than 20/200 if the macula is involved.

In AIDS patients with disseminated histoplasmosis, treatment consists of amphotericin B 0.5 to 0.8 mg/kg/day IV to a total dose of 15 mg/kg. Fluconazole 400 mg orally twice daily may also be effective.

Cryptococcosis

Cryptococcosis is a disease caused by *Cryptococcus neoformans. Cryptococcus neoformans* is recognized as a neurotropic yeast in the United States and Australia. Cutaneous cryptococcosis occurs more frequently in Europe. This yeast is common in the environment and grows well in the excreta of pigeons and most birds. Large numbers of yeast organisms can be found on dry pigeon droppings.

Pulmonary infections take place when the yeast is inhaled. Infection is also possible from basidiospores. Pulmonary lesions remain localized and may resolve spontaneously or stay encapsulated, forming fibrous nodules (cryptococcomas). Disseminated disease in immunocompromised patients is most often to the cerebromeningeal area and less frequently to the eye, skin, joints, bones, kidney, liver, and other organs. The disease is mostly asymptomatic in most healthy immunocompetent individuals, but 40% to 85% of patients have severe underlying disease or immunodeficiency.

Uveitis is attributed to simultaneous involvement of the central nervous system with cryptococcus infection. The predominant ocular manifestations include multifocal choroiditis[26] and chorioretinitis accompanied by chronic iridocyclitis. Retinal detachment may occur. Cryptococcosis occurs in patients who are immunologically compromised, especially in the older age group. The accompanying neurologic symptoms that may provide input into the nature of the ocular disease include delirium, coma, headache, and paresis of isolated muscle groups. Patients with primary cryptococcal meningitis may develop blurring of vision, retrobulbar pain, diplopia, and photophobia. The disease may occasionally be confused with Vogt-Koyanagi-Harada syndrome. One should always consider the possibility of cryptococcal infection in patients who are immunologically compromised and who present with uveitis and signs of meningitis. In general, CNS cryptococcosis is regarded as a fatal disease, and the patients may succumb to progressive meningoencephalitis. Cutaneous cryptococcosis may occur in healthy individuals and may lead to periorbital necrotizing fasciitis.[27]

Laboratory Diagnosis

Diagnosis of cryptococcal infection of the retina and choroid may be confirmed by the isolation of the *Cryptococcus neoformans* in the cerebrospinal fluid (CSF). Vitreous specimens as well as retina-choroidal parts may be obtained for the isolation of the fungus. *Cryptococcus neoformans* grows readily in culture and appears as encapsulated yeastlike cells measuring 2 to 20 μm in diameter. The cryptococcal capsular polysaccharide antigen is readily detected by latex agglutination test of CSF or serum. The yeast appears eosinophilic on hematoxylin and eosin-stained tissue sections. Pseudohyphae may be observed. Mucin stains the capsule. Direct immunofluorescence aids in confirming the diagnosis.

Treatment

The treatment of cryptococcosis includes the systemic administration of amphotericin B (see Table 6.1) and flucytosine. Miconazole, ketoconazole, fluconazole, and intraconazole have been tried. Fluconazole has been shown to be safe and effective in the treatment of cryptococcal infections.[16] It can be given intravenously 200 mg daily or 200 mg orally twice daily.

Fluconazole is effective in the treatment of cryptococcosis.[27-29] The drug has been used in the treatment of CNS cryptococcosis with ocular manifestations such as papilledema, retinitis, and optic nerve involvement.[16,28,29] The outcome of CNS cryptococcosis is poor despite the use of amphotericin B; fluconazole appears to be more effective and less toxic and was found to be effective in cases where amphotericin B had failed.[16,28,29] Fluconazole may be given for chronic suppression of cryptococcosis in patients with AIDS. Its long half-life allows the single dose administration of 200 mg orally per day. In severe cases of cryptococcosis amphotericin B may be combined with flucytosine 25 mg/kg orally every 6 hours.

Aspergillosis

Aspergillosis is a relatively rare intraocular inflammation that may occur as a result of infection with *Aspergillus tereus* or other species of aspergillus.[31-34] The organism may reach the retina or choroid through the bloodstream and may lead to disseminated choroiditis.[31-33] Aspergillus endophthalmitis may occur in drug addicts. The initial lesions may consist of multiple foci of choroiditis, which progress rapidly into a fulminant endophthalmitis requiring vitrectomy and intraocular injection of amphotericin B for the control of the infection. It should be kept in mind that intraocular aspergillosis may occur after exposure to an exogenous source of *Aspergillus* infection.

Laboratory Diagnosis

The diagnosis is confirmed by isolation of the organism from the retina or vitreous cavity.

Treatment

Patients require vitrectomy and intraocular injection of amphotericin B. The fear of aspergillus infection, especially in immunocompromised individuals, necessitates intravenous administration of amphotericin B (see Table 6.1). Organized vitreoretinal membranes may occur in the aftermath of the infection requiring surgical intervention. Vitrectomy for epiretinal membrane may be required for patients with Aspergillus infection similar to *Candida* chorioretinitis.[35]

References

1. Brooks RG: Prospective study of Candida endophthalmitis in hospitalized patients with candidemia. Arch Intern Med 1989;149(10):2226–2228.
2. Jabs DA, Green WR, Fox R, et al.: Ocular manifestations of acquired immune deficiency syndrome. Ophthalmology 1989;96:1092–1099.
3. Chess J, Kaplan S, Rubinstein A, et al.: Candida retinitis in bare lymphocyte syndrome. Ophthalmology 1986; 93(5):696–698.
4. Deutsh D, Adler S, Teller J, et al.: Endogenous candida endophthalmitis. Ann Ophthalmol 1989;21(7):260–268.
5. Despres E, Weber M, Jouart D, et al.: Candida albicans uveopapillitis: Diagnostic and therapeutic discussion a

propos of a case. Bull Soc Ophthalmol Fr 1990;1: 105–108.

6. Hayasaka S, Noda S, Setogawa T: Endogenous Candida species endophthalmitis associated with increased levels of D-Arabinitol in serum and vitreous. Am J Ophthalmol 1990;111:379–380.

7. Tollemar J, Ringden O: Early pharmakokinetic and clinical results from a noncomparative multicentre trial of Amphotericin B encapsulated in a small unilamellar liposome (AmBisome®) Drug Invest 1992;4: 232–238.

8. Grant SM, Clissold SP: Fluconazole. A review of its pharmacodynamic and pharmacokinetic properties, and therapeutic potential in superficial and systemic mycoses. Drugs 1990;39:877–916.

9. Brammer KW, Farrow PR, Faulkner JK: Pharmacokinetics and tissue penetration of fluconazole in humans. Rev Infect Dis 1990;12(Suppl 3):S318–S326.

10. Savani DV, Perfect JR, Cobo LM, Durack DT: Penetration of new azole compounds into the eye and efficacy in experimental Candida endophthalmitis. Antimicrob Agents Chemother 1987;31:6–10.

11. Abe M, Ishikawa H: Ocular penetration of fluconazole. J Eye 1991;8:1479–1481.

12. O'Day DM, Foulds G, Williams TE, et al.: Ocular uptake of fluconazole following oral administration. Arch Ophthalmol 1990;108:1006–1008.

13. Urbak SF, Degn T: Fluconazole in the treatment of Candida albicans endophthalmitis. Acta Ophthalmol 1992;70:528–529.

14. Kaneko S, Tsushima K, Aonuma H, et al.: Systemic fluconazole for endogenous fungal endophthalmitis. Jpn J Clin Ophthalmol 1991;45:1389–1392.

15. Filler SG, Crislip MA, Mayer CL, Edwards JE, Jr: Comparison of fluconazole and amphotericin B for treatment of disseminated candidiasis and endophthalmitis in rabbits. Antimicrob Agents Chemother 1991;35:288–292.

16. Agarwal A, Gupta A, Sakhuja V, et al.: Retinitis following disseminated cryptococcosis in a renal allograft recipient. Efficacy of oral fluconazole. Acta Ophthalmol 1991;69:402–405.

17. Kattan H, Pflulgfelder SC: Complications of intraocular antimicrobial agents. Int Ophthalmol Clin 1989;29: 188–194.

18. Miura Y, Kaneko S, Miura K, Watanabe I: Ocular toxicity of intravitreal fluconazole in the rabbit. Folia Ophthalmol Jpn 1992;43:35–38.

19. Hawkins BS, Ganley JP: Risk of visual impairment attributable to ocular histoplasmosis. Arch Ophthalmol 1994;112:655–666.

20. Weingeist TA, Watzke RC: Ocular involvement by Histoplasma capsulatum. Int Ophthalmol Clin 1983;23: 33–47.

21. Gutman FA: The natural course of active choroidal lesions in the presumed ocular histoplasmosis syndrome. Trans Am Ophthalmol Soc 1979;77:515–541.

22. Smith RE, Knox DL, Jensen AD: Ocular histoplasmosis: significance of asymptomatic macular scars. Arch Ophthalmol 1973;89:296–300.

23. Ryan SJ: De novo subretinal neovascularization in the histoplasmosis syndrome. Arch Ophthalmol 1976;94: 321–327.

24. Ocular histoplasmosis. JAMA 1980;243:626–627. Editorial.

25. Shields JA, Eagle RC, Barr CC, et al.: Adenocarcinoma of retinal pigment epithelium arising from a juxtapapillary histoplasmosis scar. Arch Ophthalmol 1994;112: 650–656.

26. Carney MD, Combs JL, Waschler W: Cryptococcal choroiditis. Retina 1990;10(1):27–32.

27. Doorenbos-Bot ACC, Hooymans JMM, Blanksma LJ: Periorbital necrotising fasciitis due to Cryptococcus neoformans in a healthy young man. Documenta Ophthalmol 1990;75:315–320.

28. Good CB, Leper HF: Profound papilledema due to cryptococcal meningitis in acquired immunodeficiency syndrome: Successful treatment with fluconazole. South Med J 1991;84:394–396.

29. Golnik KC, Newman SA, Wispelway B: Cryptococcal optic neuropathy in the acquired immune deficiency syndrome. J Clin Neuro-Ophthalmol 1991;11:96–103.

30. Crump JRC, Elmer SG, Elner VM, Kauffman CA: Cryptococcal endophthalmitis: case report and review. Clin Infect Dis 1992;14:1069–1073.

31. Valluri S, Moorthy RS, Liggett PE, Rao NA: Endogenous aspergillus endophthalmitis in an immunocompetent individual. Int. Ophthalmol 1993;17: 131–135.

32. Denning DW, Stevens DA: Antifungal and surgical treatment of invasive aspergillosis: review of 2121 published cases. Rev Infect Dis 1990;12:1147–1201.

33. Katz G, Winchester K, Lam S: Ocular aspergillosis isolated in the anterior chamber. Ophthalmology 1993;100: 1815–1818.

34. Bodoia RD, Kinyoun JL, Lou QL, et al.: Aspergillus necrotizing retinitis: A clinico-pathologic study and review. Retina 1989;9(3):226–231.

35. McDonald HR, De Bustros S, Sipperley JO: Vitrectomy for epiretinal membrane with Candida chorioretinitis. Ophthalmology 1990;97(4):466–469.

III

Noninfectious Diseases

Chapter 7
Autoimmune Diseases

Robert B. Nussenblatt and Khalid F. Tabbara

Several disorders present in the eye with an inflammatory response essentially directed toward the retinal vasculature. Much speculation exists as to the underlying mechanisms and to what specific antigen the inflammation is directed. Some of the entities present with overlying clinical findings, and others are relatively distinctive.

Retinal Vasculitis

We have noted over the years a group of patients who have recurrent episodes of severe inflammation centering about the retinal vasculature. These patients have posterior pole changes that appear compatible with the diagnosis of Behcet's disease, yet they do not manifest any of the other extraocular stigmata of that disorder. In our experience, these patients can have a severe inflammatory response that significantly involves the retinal vasculature. Patients have multiple explosive inflammatory episodes suggestive of Behcet's disease. These are areas of retinal infarction with hemorrhage and a swollen retina. These patients continue with severe ocular attacks, as do patients with full-blown Behcet's syndrome. If this continues unabated, the retinal disease will take on the aspect of late-stage Behcet's disease (Figures 7.1, 7.2).

What appears to distinguish these patients is that they do not go on to develop the extraocular manifestations of Behcet's disease. Most patients with Behcet's disease do not manifest ocular disease as the first sign of their disorder. Given that many of the patients with the retinal findings as just described have now been followed for an extended period, it appears that they form a separate group of patients from the Behcet group.

Diagnostic Tests

We have noted that patients presenting with this ocular picture of Behcet's disease are often human lymphocyte antigen (HLA)-B51 positive. It must be stressed that this is purely a clinical observation supported with anecdotal information, and has not yet been supported by a critical HLA study. Fluorescein angiography is very helpful in demonstrating alterations to the retinal circulation (Figure 7.3). Areas of capillary dropout as well as neovascularization can be best evaluated using this method. Auxiliary tests such as an electroretinogram may help quantify a clinical impression of severe disease, but are not particularly helpful in management of the disease.

It is interesting to speculate why these patients manifest only ocular disease, and not the systemic manifestations that are also associated with HLA-B51. The patients we have seen with this entity are white and from several different ethnic groups. It may be that various environmental or endogenous factors are needed to trigger the various manifestations of Behcet's disease, and these are not present in these patients.

Treatment

The patient's ocular course resembles that of Behcet's disease. Therefore, the treatment for their condition should be commensurate with the poten-

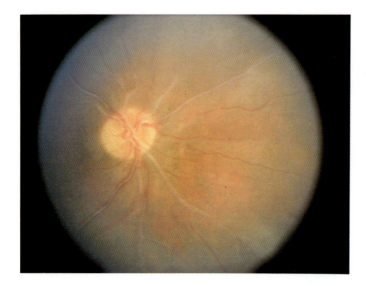

Figure 7.1. Extensive retinal vascular changes due to explosive, recurrent episodes of an ocular Behcet-like disease without systemic findings. (Courtesy of Dr. Manabu Mochizuki.)

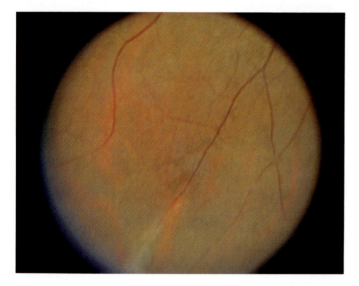

Figure 7.2. Early stages of retinal vasculitis involving the peripheral retina.

tially serious and irreversible loss of vision. We have treated a small number of these patients with cyclosporine, and have found that this approach appears to have stabilized their ocular condition.

Eales' Disease

Although he was not the first to describe this entity, Eales[1] reported in 1880 several cases of young men who had recurrent vitreal hemorrhages associated with constipation and nosebleeds. Although the latter symptoms are no longer considered part of the syndrome as we know it, a periphlebitis, particu-

larly in the retinal periphery, is an entity that has been recognized to exist.

The disorder usually occurs in young men and is rarely, if ever, seen in adults older than 45 years of age. Although the condition is usually bilateral, it usually begins unilaterally. The changes usually occur in the periphery.

It should be emphasized that this diagnosis is one of exclusion and is typically seen in young healthy individuals. Conditions such as sickle cell anemia, diabetes, and ischemic retinal disease need to be ruled out.

The treatment of the disorder centers around the use of laser ablation, if areas are recognized,

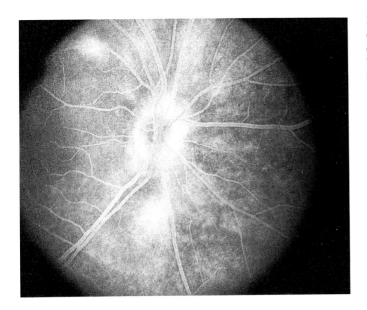

Figure 7.3. Fluorescein angiogram of fundus from a patient with diffuse retinal vasculitis unassociated with systemic disease. The areas of hyperfluorescence are at the level of the retinal vasculature.

and possibly vitrectomy for the recurrent vitreal hemorrhages.

Systemic Lupus Erythematosus

Systemic lupus erythematosus is a multisystem disease that is characterized by an alteration in a number of immunologic parameters, including a decrease in suppressor cells and autoantibody formation. The disorder appears to have a predilection for certain organs, particularly the skin, joints, hemopoietic system, central nervous system, and the kidney. The eye has been reported to be involved in 3% to 29% of cases of systemic lupus erythematosus.[2,3] The disorder can cause such ocular changes as a secondary Sjögren's syndrome and neuro-ophthalmic abnormalities; the retina can be involved as well. Cotton-wool spots and superficial hemorrhages (Figure 7.4) are the most commonly seen evidence of the retinal pathology. However, a rare complication is that of severe vaso-occlusive retinal disease. In Jabs and colleagues' excellent report of 11 patients with this disorder,[4] a whole host of retinal vascular findings were noted. In that study, the researchers found occlusion of both the central retinal artery and vein, as well as branch retinal artery. Others in the study had widespread areas of arteriolar occlusion and capillary nonperfusion. Of interest was the fact that 9 of the 13 patients developed retinal neovascularization, and 3 of 11

patients ultimately developed a retinal detachment. Approximately one-half of the eyes had a visual acuity of 20/200 or worse. Of the systemic features of the systemic lupus erythematosus, only central nervous system disease correlated with the severe retinal vaso-occlusive disease seen in these patients. In the approximately 21 other such lupus patients with severe retinal vaso-occlusive disease reported in the literature since 1947, these findings appear to be consistently seen. Rubeosis is an additional clinical finding in some of these patients. Choroidal vascular disease in patients with systemic lupus erythematosus may lead to choroiditis and multifocal serous detachment of the retinal pigment epithelium.[5,6]

Diagnostic Tests

A fluorescein angiogram must be performed on these patients to fully evaluate the extent of the disorder. In addition to the attention paid to the major vessels, the periphery needs to be scanned for evidence of capillary nonperfusion in those regions as well. Some authors have suggested that slow retinal filling times may be a feature of this disorder. Tortuosity of retinal vessels may be seen in the periphery. Ultimately, areas of perivenular cuffing become evident and the patient has an apparent periphlebitis. These changes may cause no alteration in vision, and at times come to the attention of an ophthalmologist only after the vitreal hemorrhage has blurred the vi-

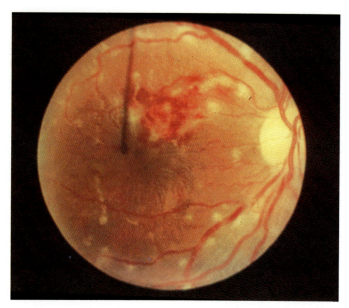

A

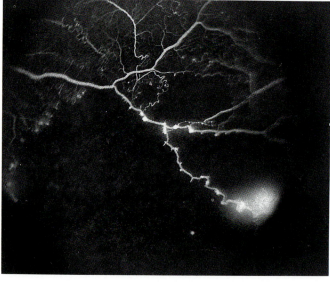

B

Figure 7.4. A, Diffuse vasculopathy of systemic lupus erythematosus. Hemorrhage and multiple never fiber layer defects (cotton-wool spots) can be seen. **B,** Fluorescein angiogram of the same patients showing dramatically large area of capillary nonperfusion as well as leakage from larger vessels.

sion. The periphlebitis appears to be randomly distributed, and does not appear to cluster around arteriovenous crossings. Ultimately venous obstruction with edema and blot hemorrhages appears. In a small number of cases this can occur near the optic disc, and the patient may have a central venous obstruction. As a consequence of the obstruction, neovascularization develops leading to recurrent vitreal hemorrhages. All of these changes occur in the absence of vitreal inflammatory activity.

The fluorescein angiogram shows areas of venous obstruction with associated areas of capillary dropout. In the later stages of the disease, there can be vitreal traction with, ultimately, retinal detachment, rubeosis iridis, and glaucoma. In some cases the course may be very mild, with a disappearance of the periphlebitis and a regression of the neovascularization.

The cause of this disease is unknown. It had been associated with previous exposure to tuberculosis.

The histopathology shows no evidence of uveitis, but shows changes compatible with a periphlebitis, and venule blood tests can be ordered to help in the diagnosis, including an ANA, anti-ssDNA antibody, anti-ribonucleoprotein antibody, anti-SM antibody, and circulating immune complexes.

The mechanism for this severe retinal vascular disorder still is only speculation, but small vessel disease attributable to lupus in other parts of the body is caused by a presumed deposition of immune complexes. Immunoglobulin deposition has been noted in the retinal vasculature.[5]

The therapeutic strategies for this type of patient must take into account many factors. For the systemic disease, frequently high-dose pulse methylprednisolone or cytotoxic therapy, possibly with the addition of a low dose of these agents for chronic use, is frequently done. From a purely ocular point of view, panretinal photocoagulation needs to be contemplated in these patients, as with anyone who has a central vein occlusion or marked capillary nonperfusion. In addition, with the neovascularization comes the risk of vitreal hemorrhage and the possible need for vitrectomy.

References

1. Eales H: Cases of retinal hemorrhage associated with epistaxis and constipation. Birmingham Med Rev 1980;9: 262–273.
2. Gold DH, Morris DA, Henkind P: Ocular findings in systemic lupus erythematosus. Br J Ophthalmol 1972;56: 800–804.
3. Lanham JG, Barrie T, Kohner E, et al.: SLE retinopathy: Evaluation by fluorescein angiography. Ann Rheum Dis 1982;41:473–478.
4. Jabs DA, Fine SL, Hochberg MC, et al.: Severe retinal vaso-occlusive disease in systemic lupus erythematosus. Arch Ophthalmol 1986;104:558–563.
5. Jabs DA, Hanneken AM, Schachat AP, Fine SL: Choroidopathy in systemic lupus erythematosus. Arch Ophthalmol 1988;106:230.
6. Carpenter MT, O'Boyle JE, Enzenauer RW, et al.: Choroiditis in systemic lupus erythematosus. Am J Ophthalmol 1994;117:535–536.

The Vogt-Koyanagi-Harada Syndrome

The Vogt-Koyanagi-Harada syndrome is a multisystem disorder affecting in particular the eye and other parts of the central nervous system as well as the ear and the skin. Various ocular features of this disorder were reported by several observers early in this century. Vogt, in 1906, and Koyanagi, in 1929, described an anterior and intermediate uveitis associated with poliosis, vitiligo, and hypoacousia. Harada, in 1926, described an inflammatory condition characterized by an exudative retinal detachment associated with a pleocytosis in the cerebrospinal fluid.[1] It was Professor Babel of Geneva, Switzerland, who suggested that these various observations were in fact features of the same disorder.[1]

Although this disorder is found worldwide, it is particularly common in Japan, where at least 8% of noninfectious uveitis cases carry this diagnosis. The disease appears to be seen frequently in South America and is not uncommon amongst certain ethnic groups in the United States, particularly those with American Indian heritage. It is a very rare entity in Scandinavia. Although more men appear to be affected in Japan, it has been our experience and that of our Brazilian confreres that this condition is more frequently seen in women.[1]

Clinical Findings (see Table 7.1)

Ocular symptoms often occur after a flulike prodrome characterized by headache, orbital pain, stiff neck, and vertigo. Sometimes the patient may be febrile. During this acute prodrome period, a spinal tap demonstrates a pleocytosis with lymphocytes and monocytes in approximately 84% of cases. The pleocytosis can disappear very rapidly, and attempts at demonstrating cells in the cerebrospinal fluid later in the course of the disease may prove fruitless. Hypo-acousia is seen in approximately 74% of cases, and the auditory alterations are mostly in the high-frequency range. Often, audiometry is needed to determine that an auditory defect is indeed present. Other typical extraocular findings in this disorder include vitiligo, alopecia, and poliosis. These changes are seen in 63% to 90% of cases. The vitiligo can be present anywhere on the body; it may encircle the lids or be found around the armpits. Patients also may complain of scalp pain when combing their hair.

The Vogt-Koyanagi-Harada syndrome is a bilateral inflammatory ocular disorder. In 94% of cases, the uveitis manifests itself in both eyes. It has been

Table 7.1. Vogt-Koyanagi-Harada Syndrome

I. DESCRIPTION

Vogt-Koyanagi-Harada (VKH) syndrome is a spectrum of disease characterized by inflammation of the uvea in both eyes. The disease may affect the posterior segment of the eye only and then is referred to as Harada's disease. When the condition is associated with anterior uveitis, vitiligo, poliosis, the condition is referred to as Vogt-Koyanagi-Harada syndrome.

II. CLINICAL PRESENTATION

A. Acute stage posterior segment retinal detachment (Nonrhegmatogenous exudative) Dalen-Fuchs nodules, edema of the optic nerve head, choroiditis

B. Sequelae

Retinal pigment epithelial changes with pigment migration, occlusion of the choriocapillaris, optic atrophy, focal retinal choroiditic scars, secondary glaucoma, phthisis bulbi

C. Symptoms
1. Prodromal symptoms: Fever, malaise, nausea
2. Other symptoms: Headaches, lethargy, neck stiffness, dysacousia, tinnitis, loss of hair, vertigo, hearing loss

D. Other Findings
1. Retinal pigment epithelial (RPE) migration, loss of RPE
2. Nonocular findings: Vitiligo, poliosis, alopecia, hearing loss

III. LABORATORY TESTS

A. Audiogram, auditory disturbances

B. Electroencephalogram (EEG) abnormal, cerebrospinal fluid shows increased proteins, pleocytosis with predominant lymphocytes, electro-oculography (EOG) and electroretinogram (ERG) changes, association with human lymphocyte antigens (HLA) BW22J and HLA BW54. HLA DRBI*0405 AND DRBI*0410.

IV. PROGNOSIS

A. 20/50 or better—50%
B. 20/200—25%
C. 20/200 or worse—25%

V. TREATMENT

A. High-dose systemic corticosteroids
B. Cyclosporine

observed by some that the disorder manifests itself more frequently in the fall and spring. Patients may present as an ocular emergency, because of a bilateral, dramatic drop in visual acuity. Among Japanese patients, one of the first findings is perilimbal vitiligo, or Segiura's sign. We have not appreciated this in the patients we have followed in the United States. The inflammation is a granulomatous inflammation with mutton fat precipitates readily seen on the corneal endothelium. Examination of the anterior chamber may show some shallowing associated with hypotony. Changes in near vision may be evident without major alterations to distant vision because of a swelling of the ciliary processes, which can be a very early finding in this disorder.[2] In new cases, the anterior segment may have a profound inflammatory reaction. Iris nodules are frequently noted (Figure 7.5). As with the anterior chamber, a severe reaction may be noted in the vitreous, sometimes making a detailed examination of the posterior segment difficult. At times, vitreous hemorrhage may obscure the view, and the source may not be evident as the inflammatory disease subsides. The posterior segment may show a shifting retinal detachment. The exudative detachment usually does not take on the appearance of that of rhegmatogenous detachment and does not usually extend back to the ora. Optic nerve swelling is quite typical, seen in 87% of cases. Frequently, diffuse retinal swelling or edema is seen posteriorly. Usually, the retinal vasculature does not appear to be remarkably affected. As the disease evolves, one typically observes deep circular lesions strewn throughout the retinal periphery. They seem to be much less frequently seen in the posterior pole. As with sympathetic ophthalmia, they are thought to be the clinical equivalent of the Dalen-Fuchs nodules that are seen histologically (Figure 7.6).

The angiogram may show several features typical of but not unique to this syndrome. Typically, multiple lesions at the level of the retinal pigment epithelium are seen. As the angiogram progresses, one sees areas of leakage from these points, frequently under an elevated retinal area (Figure 7.7). As the angiogram continues, one can see a coalescence of the multiple-areas leakage. Leakage from the optic nerve head is invariably noted as well. The lesions in the periphery may show early blockage with late staining, as is typical of active lesions below the retina. As the inflammatory disease begins to dissipate, these areas usually demonstrate a window defect phenomenon.

As the inflammatory disease subsides, several phenomena become evident. There can be a rather dramatic depigmentation of the retina, whose appearance has been called the sunset glow fundus. Subretinal scarring can take on a rather marked appearance (Figure 7.8). Clearly areas that have had

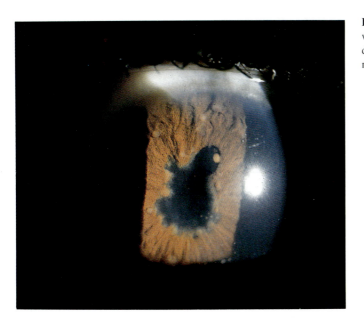

Figure 7.5. Anterior segment of patient with Vogt-Koyanagi-Harada syndrome demonstrating both Busacca and Koeppe nodules.

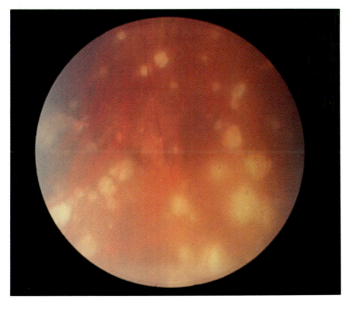

Figure 7.6. Fundus photograph of an eye from a middle-aged male who suffered a penetrating injury to contralateral eye during a hunting accident. In addition to the severe vitritis, multiple lesions formed in the peripheral retina. These are thought to be the clinical equivalent of Dalen-Fuchs nodules.

longstanding retinal detachment are at great risk, but other areas also may show these changes. A so-called "scimatar" sign has been observed, denoting a broad area of subretinal fibrosis that can extend from the optic nerve to an area temporal to the macula.

Another complication of the Vogt-Koyanagi-Harada syndrome is that of subretinal neovascularization (Figure 7.9). We think this is a poor sign when present in the peripapillary region.[2] However, eccentrically placed neovascular nets away from the macula appear to have a relatively benign course, and may even disappear with time.[3]

The diagnosis of the Vogt-Koyanagi-Harada syndrome is still a clinical one. We wish to see evidence of extraocular involvement before we are confident of the diagnosis. Statistically, we know that patients should present with extraocular findings before or at least during the ocular attack. Therefore, in addition to the uveitis as described above, we look for evidence of hearing loss, skin and hair alterations, and evidence of cen-

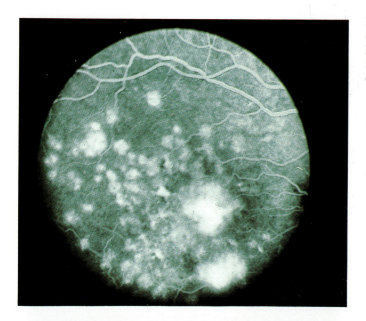

Figure 7.7. Fluorescein angiogram of fundus of patient with the Vogt-Koyanagi-Harada syndrome showing the pinpoint leakage at the level of the retinal pigment epithelium typical of this disorder.

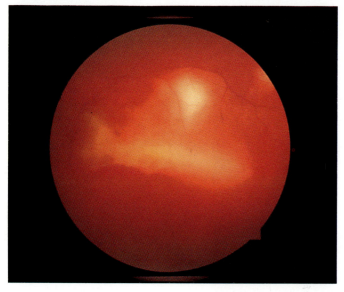

Figure 7.8. Subretinal fibrosis, sometimes in the form of a "scimitar," can be seen in patients with longstanding disease.

tral nervous system involvement, such as cells in the cerebrospinal fluid. Some colleagues use the term "Harada's disease" to designate an inflammatory condition with an exudative retinal detachment, but not extraocular findings. We have hesitated from using this term based on the philosophic concept that, because we are dealing with an entity that is purely based on the arbitrary collection of clinical findings, it is not logical to apply this definition in a less strict fashion. Because we are already uncertain as to the underlying cause of the full-blown disease, we are uncertain

that an entity resembling the original is the same or different.

The differential diagnosis includes any severe granulomatosis inflammatory disorder. Certainly a diagnosis of sarcoidosis must be entertained, particularly if there is a lack of extraocular findings in the patient. Sympathetic ophthalmia so closely resembles this entity that it must always be considered, particularly when a history of trauma or multiple ocular surgeries is part of the history. If seen late in its course, and if it has not been aggressively treated, the eyes may have a

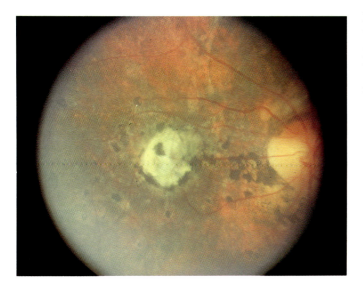

Figure 7.9. Fundus photograph of patient with longstanding Vogt-Koyanagi-Harada syndrome that has become quiescent. Marked pigment disturbances are seen. A subretinal scar secondary to neovascularization is evident as well under the macula.

residual detachment with little inflammatory disease, thereby mimicking the findings in the uveal effusion syndrome.

Histology and Laboratory Tests

The histologic appearance of the Vogt-Koyanagi-Harada syndrome strongly resembles that seen in sympathetic ophthalmia, with, however, some differences. In this syndrome, one usually sees a scarring of the choriocapillaris, whereas there is a so-called "sparing" of this region in sympathetic ophthalmia. In the Vogt-Koyanagi-Harada syndrome, there is a profound loss of pigment throughout all layers of the choroid, as well as the retinal pigment epithelium.

Immunologic testing has shown rather distinct responses relating to patients with this disorder. An association with HLA-DR4 and DQ3 has been seen in American patients, and DR53 was seen in Japanese patients. Recent studies have shown a strong association between VKH and DRBI*0405 and DRBI*0410. Immunologic testing has also revealed that these patients have cytotoxic T cells that have been sensitized against antigens presumed to be on the surface of pigmented cells.[4] Hence there is a presumed link between skin, eye, and ear; these organs all have pigmented cells.

Therapy

The treatment of choice for this disorder is with systemic corticosteroids. In the acute situation, in which there is an exudative detachment and a dramatic loss of vision, the dosage of the systemic corticosteriods is particularly high, for example, 100 to 200 mg prednisone. An alternative approach for particularly difficult cases is to administer 250 mg methylprednisolone intravenously (or 1 g daily) for 3 days, assuming that there are no medical contraindications. After this initially high dosage, usually prednisone is given orally at a dosage of 1 mg/kg/day. The duration of therapy must be individualized, with continued vigilance against recurrences. Although the literature speaks of this disorder as being self-limited, and therapy can be given for a relatively short duration, we have found that a significantly large number of patients in fact have ongoing chronic inflammatory disease. Generally, if we need to treat a patient with relatively high doses of daily prednisone (30 mg or more) for a period that is longer than 3 to 4 months, we will consider alternative medications. Cytotoxic agents have not been widely used for the treatment of this disorder in the United States. However, in Latin America, this approach to therapy is used with reasonably good success.[5] We have used cyclosporine in the treatment of steroid-resistant cases with success.[6] A recent report in the Japanese literature reports control of this disorder with a combination of cyclosporine and systemic steroid in a patient previously requiring 200 mg prednisone to control his disease.[7]

Treatment of the subretinal membranes with laser is a difficult question. Certainly subretinal nets approaching the macular region should be aggressively treated. However, the more eccentrically placed nets probably can be watched, because some disappear on their own accord when adequate antiinflammatory/immunosuppressive therapy is administered.

References

1. Nussenblatt RB, Palestine AG: The Vogt-Koyanagi-Harada syndrome, in Uveitis: Fundamentals and Clinical Practice. Chicago: Yearbook Medical Publishers Inc., 1989, 274–290.
2. Kimura R, Kasai M, Shoji K, et al.: Swollen ciliary processes as an initial symptom in Vogt-Koyanagi-Harada syndrome. Arch Ophthalmol 1983;95:402–403.
3. Davis JL, Palestine AG, Nussenblatt RB: Neovascularization in uveitis. Ophthalmology 1988;95(Suppl):171.
4. Maezawa N, Yano A: Requirement of 1a-positive nylon wool adherent cells for the activation of cytotoxic T lymphocytes specific for melanocyte-associated antigens in patients with Vogt-Koyanagi-Harada's disease. Jpn J Ophthalmol 1988;32:348–357.
5. Orefice F: Syndrome Vogt-Koyanagi-Harada, in: Uveitis. Conselho Brasileiro de Oftalmologia. F. Orefice and Rubens Belfort Jr (eds.). Roca, Sao Paolo, 1987:299.
6. Nussenblatt RB, Palestine AG, Chan CC: Cyclosporin A therapy in the treatment of intraocular inflammatory disease resistant to systemic corticosteroids and cytotoxic agents. Am J Ophthalmol 1983;96:275–282.
7. Wakatsuki Y, Kogure M, Takahashi Y, et al.: The combination therapy of cyclosporin A and steroid in the severe case of Vogt-Koyanagi-Harada's disease. Jpn J Ophthalmol 1988;32:358–360.

Sympathetic Ophthalmia

Sympathetic ophthalmia is probably the best known of the intraocular inflammatory conditions to our medical colleagues outside the specialty of ophthalmology. The number of patients with this disorder per year is probably fairly small. The fear of potential bilateral blindness, however, is clearly very great. The disorder was known to the ancients, but it was MacKenzie in the middle of the last century who coined the term "sympathetic ophthalmia" and described the clinical condition.

Sympathetic ophthalmia is a bilateral granulomatous uveitis that follows penetrating trauma to the globe, whether accidental or from a surgical intervention. The trauma to one eye incites an inflammatory reaction in the other eye. Sympathetic ophthalmia may occur several days to several decades after the original penetrating injury. More than 80% of the cases become apparent clinically by 3 months after the penetrating wound. It has been estimated that this disorder appears in approximately 0.2% to 0.5% of cases of accidental penetrating trauma. It has been estimated that the incidence after surgery is 10 cases per 100,000. Sympathetic ophthalmia has been reported after many different types of surgical procedures. Earlier procedures for the treatment of glaucoma, in which an iris "wick" was intentionally created, appeared to have a relatively high incidence of the disease. However, it appears that multiple intraocular procedures on the same eye increase the potential for the development of the disorder. Of particular note is the risk after successive vitrectomies and other manipulations for retinal detachment.

Clinical Findings

Biomicroscopic evaluation may disclose a granulomatous response in the anterior chamber. Mutton fat keratitic precipitates may be noted on the endothelial surface of the cornea. At times the anterior chamber reaction may be relatively unimportant. The vitreous reaction can be quite marked, with large numbers of cells and haze. The posterior segment manifests rather typical lesions. These circular whitish-creamy lesions may be found strewn throughout the fundus, usually situated outside of the temporal arcade. Sometimes these lesions can become confluent. On close examination during the active phase of the disease, these lesions appear to have substance, and are deep to the retina. Eventually they appear to become flat and atrophic and may or may not have pigment migrating to the edge. These lesions are thought to be the clinical equivalent of the Dalen-Fuchs nodule, a histologic diagnosis. Optic nerve edema can be a very prominent feature of the posterior segment disease as well. Although this disorder is classically described as affecting the choroid, approximately 50% of the eyes have some sort of retinal involvement, whether a retinal vasculitis or marked destruction of the photoreceptors.[1]

Classically described as purely an ocular disorder, there can be extraocular findings, albeit rarely so, unlike those seen in the Vogt-Koyanagi-Harada syndrome, in which these findings are important in establishing the diagnosis. However, in sympathetic ophthalmia, cells in the cerebrospinal fluid, hearing difficulties, and even vitiligo and poliosis have been observed. Two ocular conditions have been associated with sympathetic ophthalmia. Phacoanaphylaxis occurs in 23% to 46% of cases of sympathetic ophthalmia. Melanoma of the choroid is also associated with this disorder. In one study, this tumor was found in seven of four hundred cases of sympathetic ophthalmia studied histologically at the Armed Forces Institute of Pathology.[2] Such a finding suggests extrascleral spread of the tumor, creating in essence a penetrating wound.

The differential diagnosis in terms of the clinical appearance of sympathetic ophthalmia includes several granulomatous conditions, including sarcoidosis and the Vogt-Koyanagi-Harada syndrome. Milder inflammatory responses after a penetrating injury have mimicked acute multifocal placoid pigment epitheliopathy (AMPPE).

The resultant effects of the ongoing inflammation seen in this disease are quite variable, depending considerably on the severity of the inflammatory response as well as on the efficacy of the treatment. With a severe anterior segment inflammation, one may see the development of a secondary glaucoma. Cataract is a very common result of this inflammatory condition. Although considered purely a choroidal condition, retinal changes that can be documented with electrophysiologic testing can be seen and may be severe. Optic nerve atrophy may be the result of severe retinal involvement.

The diagnosis of sympathetic ophthalmia is relatively straightforward when a bilateral inflammatory condition appears after penetrating trauma. Other clinical presentations may be considerably more subtle, however, with the diagnosis most difficult to make. This is particularly true in cases after multiple surgical procedures for retinal disease, and particularly if there has been a history of uveitis previously. One then has to turn to the list of characteristics of the disorder and attempt to rule out other conditions. In cases of phacoanaphylaxis, one sees active inflammation in only one eye at a time (even if bilateral),[3] whereas in cases of sympathetic ophthalmia one expects to see bilaterally active disease.

Diagnostic Tests

The tests currently available permit one to judge the severity of the condition but do not really help in di-

agnosing the condition, which is based solely on the clinical presentation and events, with subsequent histologic confirmation.

Fluorescein angiography can help enormously in the evaluation of posterior segment. During the active period of the disease, one can see early blockage with late staining of the active, deep, circular lesions. The retinal vessels may also demonstrate late staining, and there can be optic nerve leakage. In our experience, cystoid macular edema is an unusual finding in these patients. With time, the areas corresponding to Dalen-Fuchs nodules become atrophic and show simply as a window defect. The electroretinogram and electrooculogram can be helpful in assessing the degree of damage. In cases with good central vision, one can consider performing repeat visual field testing to evaluate the extent and progression of disease.

The histologic description of this disorder was most adequately reported by the early portion of this century, particularly by Fuchs.[4] The classic description centers around to profound changes that are noted in the choroid. Classically, the choroid is markedly thickened (Figure 7.10). This thickening is caused by a dramatic influx of lymphocytes that surround focal areas of nonnecrotic granulomatous lesions. Early in the course of the disease, eosinophils can be noted, and B cells can be identified in the periphery of the choroid. However, immunohistologic staining techniques have clearly identified the predominant cell in the choroid to be the T cell. Indeed, the T cell subtype seen during the acute periods of the disease is the CD4+ subtype, those cells associated with helper/inducer functions. As the disease proceeds, there is a change in the T cell subtype that is present. The CD8+subtype, those associated with suppressor/cytotoxic functions, are found with increasing frequency. The Dalen-Fuchs nodule, with its epithelioid cells, which are typical but not pathognomonic of the disease, is made up of altered retinal pigment epithelial cells, macrophages, and some T cells (Figure 7.11). It appears that early on in the disease, the Dalen-Fuchs nodules that form are relatively small, and primarily contain retinal pigment epithelial cells and T cells.

The underlying mechanism that leads to this disorder is still unknown. Human lymphocyte antigen (HLA) typing suggests at least some genetic predisposition, but the association with HLA-ALL

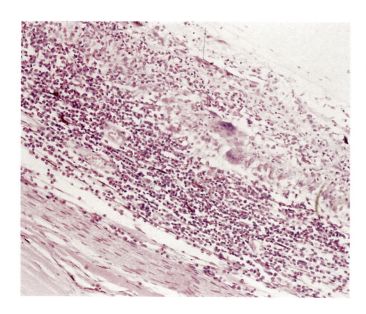

Figure 7.10. The histologic appearance of sympathetic ophthalmia classically shows a markedly thickened choroid, populated in large part by CD4+ T cells during the early portion of the disease course.

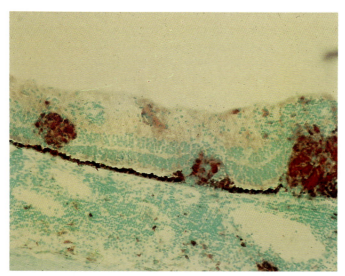

Figure 7.11. Immunologic staining of the Dalen-Fuchs nodules in this case of sympathetic ophthalmia demonstrates that most of the cells present are of macrophage origin.

(Acute Lymphocytic Leukemia) is relatively weak as compared with other HLA-associated diseases. An infectious process has been suggested for some time, although there is little to support this concept. However, that this is an autoimmune driven disorder is a hypothesis that has been proposed for many years. More recently, it has been suggested that the offending antigens may be found in the retina. Theories concerning the initiating process of this disorder must clearly take into consideration the penetrating injury, which alters the unique way that the eye processes antigen, because normally no lymphatics are present. With a penetrating injury, the lymphatic system can potentially play a role in ocular drainage. Additionally, injury may introduce adjuvants that could help in causing a more severe local response, which overwhelms the normal suppressor mechanisms that are present.

Treatment

A discussion of the treatment of this disorder must begin with the question of the role of enucleation. It has been known since the last century that removal of the injured eye before the expression of disease in the contralateral eye essentially cures this disease. Recent observations suggest that enucleation may even have a salutary effect on the course of the disease, even up to 2 weeks after the expression of the bilateral disease. We do not recommend enucleation of the injured eye except if the eye is so injured that a primary closure of the wound would be impossible. It should be remembered that the probability of developing this disease is quite small, and it appears that medical therapy is reasonably effective in treating this disorder.

In some cases, no therapy need be given immediately, because patients may retain good vision in spite of the ongoing inflammation. We treat the inflammatory disease with oral prednisone, beginning therapy with 1 to 1½ mg/kg. We usually do not use topical steroids alone, but would certainly use them in conjunction with systemic therapy to help control a severe anterior inflammatory response. Once control of the disease has been obtained, then a slow decrease in use of the steroid can be entertained, with the hope that the patient could tolerate prednisone by mouth at a dosage of 15 to 25 mg per day. We might contemplate therapy for 1 year.

If, however, a chronically high dose of prednisone is needed to control the ongoing inflammatory disease, we then turn to cyclosporine, with a starting oral dose usually of 5 mg/kg/day. Frequently we give the drug in conjunction with a relatively small amount of prednisone, from 10 to 20 mg/day. A long period of therapy is also contemplated using this approach. It is imperative that the treating physician follow the guideline for cyclosporine therapy that have been outlined.[5] As a third alternative, we might consider the use of cytotoxic agents. Certainly one can find reports in the literature of their effectiveness in this condition.[6] However, because of the long-term side effects of these agents, we prefer to reserve them for the last, when no other modality has worked.

References

1. Croxatto JO, Rao NA, McLean IW, et al.: A typical histopathologic features in sympathetic ophthalmia: A study of a hundred cases. Int Ophthalmol 1981;3: 129–135.
2. Romaine H: Malignant melanoma of the choroid with sympathetic ophthalmia. Arch Ophthalmol 1949;42: 102–103.
3. de Veer JA: Bilateral endopthalmitis phacoanaphylactica. Arch Ophthalmol 1953;49:607–632.
4. Fuchs E: Textbook of Ophthalmology. Translated by A. Duane. Philadelphia: J.B. Lippincott, 1911.
5. BenEzra D, Nussenblatt RB, Timonen P: Optimal use of sandimmun in endogenous uveitis. Berlin: Springer-Verlag, 1988.
6. Wong VG: Immunosuppressive therapy of ocular inflammatory disease. Arch Ophthalmol 1969;81:628–637.

Other Autoimmune Disorders

Other conditions deserve mention here because of the potentially severe effects they may have on the posterior segment. An autoimmune cause for these conditions is still highly speculative.

Pars Planitis

This condition is usually classified as belonging to the intermediate uveitis group. A marked effect on the retinal vasculature may be seen. The entity usually appears in the teenage years and into early adulthood. It is a bilateral condition seen in both sexes. It is characterized by an inflammatory response, which can be observed in the vitreous. Additionally, a collection of exudative material is seen, sometimes only with scleral depression, over the peripheral retina and pars plana. More recent evidence suggests that it appears to be a condition of the peripheral retina. These peripheral retinal exudates are commonly referred to as snowbanks, and they tend to be present inferiorly, although they can at times completely encircle the retina.

Marked changes in the retinal vasculature can be appreciated. Cystoid macular edema appears to be the major cause for a decrease in visual acuity in these patients. Additionally, the peripheral retina may show extensive alterations to its peripheral vasculature, with vascular sheathing and attenuation. In a series of drawings published by Brockhorst,[1] depicting such changes, the result may be a markedly atrophic retina, presumably caused by the retinal vascular compromise that has occurred as a result of this disorder.

Peripheral retina neovascularization, particularly from a point within the snowbank, is a complication that in our experience occurs more frequently in children. Recurrent vitreal hemorrhage may ensue, with the risk of vitreal traction ultimately leading to a retinal detachment.

Several conditions may simulate this condition. Sarcoidosis is known to present with an intraocular inflammatory condition similar to pars planitis. In our experience, the peripheral vascular changes may be quite similar, but the exudative lesions usually do not appear as a simple wide band extending for 180° around the peripheral retina. They tend to form as "puffballs" strewn throughout the periphery. Additionally, a uniocular presentation of pars planitis must make the observer at least pause and consider another diagnosis. *Toxocara canis* can present as a lesion in the extreme periphery, and only in one eye. A bandlike radial area of inflammation can also be attributable to ocular toxoplasmosis. Peripheral uveitis has been associated with multiple sclerosis, although it is a minority of patients with this entity that manifest this systemic disease.

There has been an ongoing debate as to whether pars planitis is distinct from intermediate uveitis without snowbanks. Henderly and colleagues[2] have reported their experience with pars planitis and have noted that although in one eye the typical snowbanks of this entity may be seen, the contralateral eye may not have these lesion, only an intermediate uveitis with vitreal cells and haze.

Tests and Pathophysiology

Fluorescein angiography is an important adjunct in helping to follow the clinical course of these patients. Evidence of macular edema on the angiogram is an important confirmatory test to document a loss of vision (Figure 7.12). Fluorescein angioscopy also may be performed if an area of focal retinal neovascularization in the periphery is suspected, and it is too far in the periphery to photograph.

Although HLA typing has been performed in these patients, we have not found a linkage with a specific antigen (unpublished results). *In vitro* testing of immune cells from pars planitis patients has shown that some of them have *in vitro* cell-mediated responses to the S-antigen. However, the number of S-antigen responders is moderate[4] as compared with other conditions, and therefore it seems doubtful that this is an underlying cause rather than a result of the retinal destruction that has occurred.

A few patients with this condition have been examined histologically. The peripheral retina demonstrates a fibroglial proliferation, particularly by Müller cells (Figure 7.13). There are also activated T cells and B cells present within this inflammatory reaction. The antigen to which these cells are responding still remains unknown.

Therapy

Observation of the condition can be considered if the visual acuity is 20/40 or better. Corticosteroids, given either systematically or periocularly, should be considered as a mode of therapy. Topical therapy is not effective for the posterior segment changes if the patient is phakic. Cryotherapy has been debated

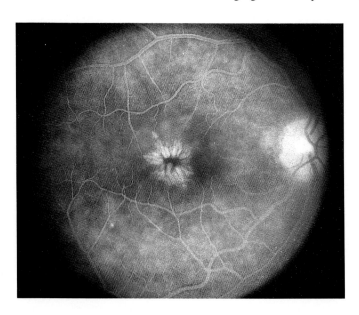

Figure 7.12. Cystoid macular edema in a patient with pars planitis. The edema can be very persistent even with the diminution of the inflammatory activity in the vitreous.

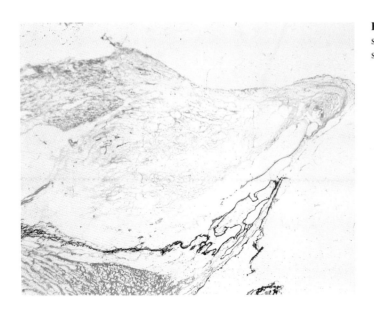

Figure 7.13. Histopathologic picture of a snowbank in an eye with pars planitis, showing the fibrous nature of the lesion.

as a possible curative therapeutic mode to these patients.[5] In our hands, cryotherapy to the area of snowbank is frequently effective in children with this condition. It is palliative rather than curative, however, but sometimes for an extended period. The snowbank often is seen to re-form, however, at times posterior to the area of cryoablation.

Neovascularization within the snowbank needs to be treated; cryotherapy appears to be the treatment of choice. Cyclosporine and cytotoxic agents have been used, but they should be considered for those severe cases that cannot be controlled with steroid. We still do not know how to differentiate between those patients who will have a benign course and those who will continue to progress, developing severe retinal vascular changes.

Subretinal Fibrosis and Uveitis Syndrome

This entity was probably first described as a single case by Fuchs in his atlas of retinal diseases.[8] However, we had an opportunity to observe several patients with this entity, giving us an idea as to its natural course.[3]

Clinical Presentation

This entity has been seen only in women, both white and black. Patients have a moderate degree of cells and haze in their vitreous. The fundus initially shows small patches of subretinal fibrosis. Initially,

because of their size, it may be difficult to make the diagnosis. The lesions are yellow in color and are underneath the retina (Figure 7.14). The inflammatory response in the vitreous is diffuse and does not center around the lesions themselves. Cystoid macular edema may or may not be an associated finding. As time goes on, one may see an enlarging of these lesions and ultimately a confluence. As long as the macular region is not involved, the patient usually enjoys good vision. The clinical course of this entity seems to be quite variable, and the factors that cause progression are not known. If the disease progresses through the macula, good vision will be lost.

It is important to rule out several conditions that could possibly mimic the subretinal fibrosis with uveitis syndrome. Sarcoidosis can induce subretinal fibrosis, as can the Vogt-Koyanagi-Harada syndrome. A longstanding retinal detachment also may induce subretinal fibrotic changes. The lesions in these disorders show considerably more perturbation of the retinal pigment epithelial layer and rarely are as confluent and large as are the lesions seen in the subretinal fibrosis with uveitis syndrome. Additionally, these subretinal lesions have a far more yellow appearance.

Diagnostic Tests

We are not aware of any tests that can help the clinician in making the diagnosis of this entity. Too few cases have been seen to do HLA typing, and the var-

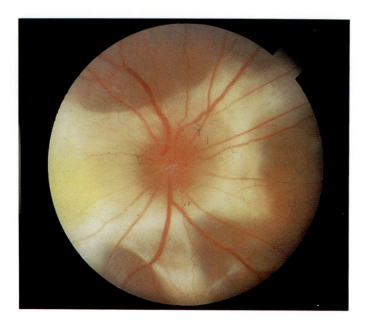

Figure 7.14. Fundus photograph of an eye with subretinal fibrosis with uveitis syndrome.

ious racial ancestries of these patients further complicate the issue. Visual field testing may show a dense scotoma in areas of retinal involvement. For areas affected by these lesions, fluorescein angiography may show window defects early on in the course of the disease, whereas late in the disease one can expect to see blockage of dye (Figure 7.15).

Two eyes with this condition have been studied. The histopathologic changes show that the retina overlying these deep lesions is atrophic.[6,7] The inflammatory infiltrate below the retina is made up primarily of B cells, with deposition of compliment at the leading edge. Additionally, there was destruction of the retinal pigment epithelial (RPE) layer, with remaining RPE cells surrounded by a sea of fibrotic or glial material. Therefore, this entity appears to be fundamentally different from the predominantly T-cell–mediated disorders such as the Vogt-Koyanagi-Harada syndrome, sarcoidosis, and sympathetic ophthalmia.

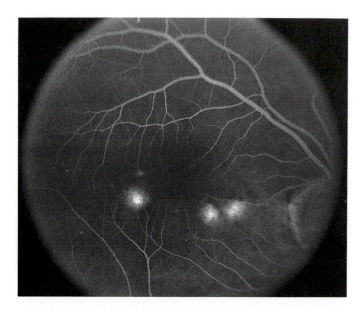

Figure 7.15. Fluorescein angiogram of an eye with subretinal fibrosis with uveitis syndrome. Note the numerous areas of hyperfluorescence that are at the level of the retinal pigment epithelium.

Therapy

This disorder has been an especially perplexing disease to treat. Corticosteroids do not seem to be particularly effective, based on the histology, but is what we would expect of cyclosporine, which has its effect primarily on T cells. We have recently seen a possibly positive response to therapy with azathioprine (Imuran®) (Burroughs Wellcome, Research Triangle Park, NC). However, not enough patients have been treated with any particular approach to enable a definitive statement to be made.

References

1. Brockhurst RJ, Schepens CL, Okamura ID: Uveitis II Peripheral uveitis: Clinical description, complications, and differential diagnosis. Am J Ophthalmol 1960;49: 1257–1266.
2. Henderly DE, Haymond RS, Rao NA, et al.: The significance of the pars plana exudate in pars planitis. Am J Ophthalmol 1987;103:669–671.
3. Palestine AG, Nussenblatt RB, Parver LM, et al.: Progressive subretinal fibrosis and uveitis. Br J Ophthalmol 1984;68:667–673.
4. de Smet MD, Yamamoto JH, Mochizuki M, et al.: Cellular immune responses of patients with uveitis to retinal antigens and their fragments. Am J Ophthalmol 1990; 110:135–142.
5. Aaberg TM, Cesarz TJ, Flicklinger RR: Treatment of pars planitis with cryotherapy. Surv Ophthalmol 1977;22: 125–129.
6. Palestine AG, Nussenblatt RB, Chan CC, et al.: Histopathology of the subretinal fibrosis and uveitis syndrome. Ophthalmology 1985;92:838–844.
7. Kin MK, Chan CC, Belfort R Jr, et al.: Histopathologic and immunohistopathologic features of subretinal fibrosis and uveitis syndrome. Am J Ophthalmol 1987;104: 15–23.
8. Fuchs E: Textbook of Ophthalmology. Translated by A. Duane. Philadelphia: J.B. Lippincott, 1911.

Birdshot Retinochoroidopathy

Birdshot retinochoroidopathy is an entity described by Ryan and Maumenee,[1] and soon after by Gass,[2] who used the name "vitiliginous choroidopathy." It is an entity that appears to be more important than the number of patients with the disorder, because of its exceptionally strong human lymphocyte antigen (HLA) association and the questions of retinal autoimmunity. It is relatively commonly seen in patients from France and the Benelux countries, suggesting once again a rather unique genetically restricted entity.

Signs and Symptoms

Birdshot retinochoroidopathy typically has its onset in patients who are usually somewhat older, with the disorder beginning in the fourth and fifth decades, whereas the onset of other uveitic conditions often occurs at an earlier age. Gass reported that vitiligo is regularly seen in these patients; hence, the name vitiliginous choroidopathy. We have not noticed this in our patients. It is a bilateral condition found in both men and women. In our experience, it is found essentially in patients of middle and northern European heritage. We have not observed this entity in black Americans nor in Hispanics. The disease may have an insidious onset, with the patient noting floaters. Ultimately there is a painless decrease in vision in one or both of the eyes.

An ocular examination usually demonstrates little or no inflammatory reaction in the anterior chamber. Although cataracts certainly may be seen in this entity, it has appeared later in the course of the disorder. The vitreous has both cells and haze, but usually not severely enough to markedly hamper an examination of the posterior segment. Examination of the posterior segment indicates several findings important in the diagnosis. Round-oval, cream-white colored lesions are seen strewn throughout the fundus (Figure 7.16). Their distribution can take on several forms.[3] These lesions are usually approximately one-third of a disc diameter or larger. They usually do not have particularly well-defined borders, and they appear to be deep to the retina, perhaps at the level of the RPE or choriocapillaris. The lesions sometimes can appear to be very subtle, particularly in a blond fundus, and the indirect ophthalmoscope is sometimes the best way to detect these lesions. During the active phase of the disease, the white-cream–colored lesions may appear to have some substance to them. As the disease progresses, the lesions may change in a variety of ways, from disappearing to leaving atrophic circular spots. The periphery of the retina and pars plana show no evidence of snowbanking. The most common reason for the decrease in vision is that of macular edema. Additionally, retinal vascular involvement can be

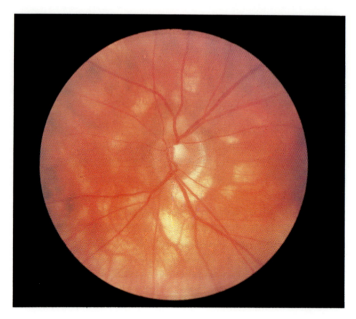

Figure 7.16. Multiple cream-colored lesions of birdshot retinochoroidopathy in an HLA-A29–positive man with cystoid macular edema.

prominent, as best seen with a fluorescein angiogram, but sometimes manifesting as a branch vein occlusion (Table 7.2).

As the disease progresses, its chronic inflammatory nature usually becomes quite evident. Even in those individuals who maintain good visual acuity, an ongoing vitreal response can be quite striking. In addition, in the late stage of the disease, the RPE may appear to lose its pigment, with the result being a very blond, almost albino-appearing fundus (Figure 7.17). As with any patient who has ongoing chronic uveitis, there is a risk of subretinal neovascularization. This complication appears to occur less frequently in this disorder than in others that resemble this disease clinically, such as the multifocal choroiditis syndrome, reviewed by Dreyer and Gass.[4] In spite of no major flare-ups, and no macular edema, the patient may face a slow decrease in vision, presumably caused by a degenerative process that had been initiated by the inflammatory process.

The differential diagnosis in essence includes disorders that can appear with multiple white lesions in the posterior segment. One important consideration is the multifocal choroiditis syndrome, as reviewed by Dreyer and Gass.[4] Sarcoidosis also may have a clinical appearance not dissimilar to birdshot retinochoroidopathy. The cream-colored lesions of birdshot retinochoroidopathy have a different appearance than they do in the entities mentioned. Here, the lesions appear poorly circumscribed and the fluorescein angiogram may be

Table 7.2. Pertinent Clinical Aspects of Birdshot Retinochoroidopathy

Anterior chamber with minimal or no inflammation
Vitreous cells with some haze
Deep, circular cream-colored lesions usually seen from the posterior pole to the vortex veins, sometimes hard to detect, requiring an indirect ophthalmoscope
Bilateral disease
Fluorescein angiogram shows evidence of retinal vascular leakage and cystoid macular edema. The birdshot lesions may or may not be seen on the angiogram.

quite helpful as well (see the following discussion and Figure 7.18).

Pathogenesis

The information that has been gathered concerning this disorder strongly suggests that autoimmunity plays an important if not a dominant role. Several observations point to this. The first is the strong association of HLA-A29 and birdshot retinochoroidopathy, corroborated by several groups.[5–7] The relative risk calculated for this antigen and this disorder ranges from 50 to 100, making it one of the most important HLA associations to date. This genetic restriction is underlined by the fact that the disease occurs perhaps exclusively in whites from France and the Benelux countries. A second point is the large number of birdshot retinochoroidopathy patients who demonstrate *in vitro* cell-mediated re-

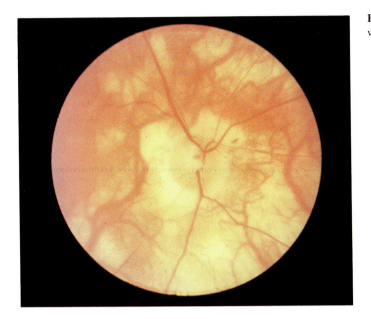

Figure 7.17. "Blond" fundus of patient with inactive birdshot retinochoroidopathy.

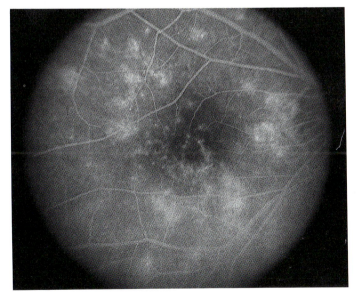

Figure 7.18. Fluorescein angiogram of fundus from patient shown in Figure 7.16. Here the lesions do appear as areas of hyperfluorescence, but frequently they do not appear on the angiogram.

sponses to the retinal S-antigen.[5] A final point would be the comparisons with this entity that have been examined. The disorder, both clinically and histologically, is quite suggestive of a disease seen in nonhuman primates who have experimentally induced S-antigen uveoretinitis.

One may speculate that patients with birdshot retinochoroidopathy have a genetic predisposition to develop an ocular autoimmune process. This could be because of an alteration in the normal suppressor mechanisms that are usually in play. Other possible mechanisms can be intoned as well. This includes the abnormal expression of HLA antigens on resident ocular cells, thereby permitting their playing an increased role in initiating an immune response, as has been suggested in a hypothesis by Botazzo and colleagues.[8]

Laboratory Testing

Clinical judgment still remains the crucial factor in determining the diagnosis of birdshot retinochoroidopathy. In this entity, however, the observer can gain important supportive information. HLA typing appears to be an important component to the work-up of a patient suspected to have this disorder. We expect to see that the patient in question is HLA-A29 positive. If not, we seriously reconsider our diagnosis. In addition, we test patients for evidence of cell-mediated responses to the retinal S-antigen, because a very high percentage of birdshot patients also demonstrate this response. This test is difficult to obtain, because it requires a separation of lymphocytes and placing them in culture.

A fluorescein angiogram is helpful in documenting the degree of macular edema, as well as the involvement of the retinal vessels, which can be a very prominent part of the disorder. Additionally, it is important to be vigilant for the appearance of subretinal neovascularization, which, although less commonly seen in this entity than in the multifocal choroiditis syndrome, can still occur. A curious finding is that the creamy-white lesions cannot always be found on fluorescein angiography, as was initially observed by Gass.[2] We concur to a degree. In some cases we have seen early blockage and late staining of the lesions (see Figure 7.18). Whether this represents a different stage of the lesions remains to be determined. Other tests, such as an electroretinogram, also can be helpful in determining the extent of the disease, which can cause rather profound changes in retinal function.

Therapy

The ideal therapeutic approach to patients with birdshot retinochoroidopathy still remains elusive. We frequently see patients with this disorder who maintain good visual acuity in both eyes. We have elected not to treat these patients. Whether this approach in the long term is a wise one needs further study. It is necessary to balance the effectiveness of immunosuppressive therapy with its side effects, however.

With a decrease in visual acuity bilaterally to a level below 20/40, one should consider beginning prednisone therapy. Topical therapy has no real place in the therapy of this disorder because the anterior segment is at best mildly inflamed. For unilateral decreases in visual acuity, we attempt a series of periocular steroid injections. As with other disorders requiring systemic steroid therapy, one must clearly attempt to reduce the dosage to the lowest level yielding acceptable vision. The effectiveness of this mode of therapy has never been evaluated in a quantified manner. Some observers suggest that the long-term visual prospects of birdshot chorioretinopathy patients is not good. Whether this observation will hold true or not, it has been our experience that often the treatment of these patients is a long-term endeavor, and frequently modalities other than systemic steroids need to be considered. We have used cyclosporine in patients with this entity in whom systemic steroids could not be continued, either because of a poor therapeutic effect or because of secondary effects. As of this writing, we will begin therapy with a dosage of 5 mg/kg/day of cyclosporine, usually combined with a relatively small amount of prednisone, from 10 to 15 mg per day.[9] We would begin cyclosporine only for those individuals in whom there is no well-controlled hypertension and also no evidence of renal disease. Although we have the opportunity to perform more detailed renal testing, we believe that at least a creatinine clearance should be performed, because changes in this test may reflect alterations in renal function attributable to cyclosporine before there are any changes in the serum creatinine. Renal alterations and hypertension have been the two major unwanted secondary effects of cyclosporine therapy. We are not aware of an extensive experience using cytotoxic agents in the treatment of this disorder. A small number of anecdotal observations have not been exceptionally positive, but if our understanding of this disorder is correct, this approach to therapy seems to be reasonable. However, increased surveillance of the patient is clearly called for if such a therapeutic route is chosen. One potential problem with this approach is that birdshot retinochoroidopathy patients frequently need to be treated for an extended period, an approach that could increase the possibility of secondary side effects caused by the cytotoxic agents.

Cataract formation is not seen frequently in these patients. In our experience many develop these fairly late in the course of their disease. When this is the case, we have elected, after discussion with the patient, to implant an intraocular lens, with reasonably good results.

References

1. Ryan SJ, Maumenee AE: Birdshot retinochoroidopathy. Am J Ophthalmol 1980;89:31–45.
2. Gass JDM: Vitiliginous chorioretinitis. Arch Ophthalmol 1981;99:1778–1787.
3. Fuerst DJ, Tessler HH, Fishman GA, et al.: Birdshot retinochoroidopathy. Arch Ophthalmol 1984;102:214–219.
4. Dreyer RF, Gass JDM: Multifocal choroiditis and panuveitis. Arch Ophthalmol 1984;102:1776–1784.
5. Nussenblatt RB, Mittal KK, Ryan SJ, et al.: Birdshot retinochoroidopathy associated with HLA-A29 antigen and immune responsiveness to retinal S-antigen. Am J Ophthalmol 1982;94:147–158.
6. Baarsma GS, Kijlstra A, Oosterhuis JA, et al.: Association of birdshot retinochoroidopathy and HLA-A29 antigen. Doc Ophthalmol 1986;61:267–269.
7. Le Hoang P, Donnefort N, Foucault C, et al.: Association between HLA A29 antigen and birdshot retinochoroidopathy. Proceedings of the XXVth International Congress of Ophthalmol (Rome). Acta XXV Concilium 1986:45–46.
8. Botazzo GF, Pujol-Borrell R, Hanafusa T, et al.: Role of aberrant HLA-DR expression and antigen presentation in induction of endocrine autoimmunity. Lancet 1983;2:1115–1119.
9. BenEzra D, Nussenblatt RB, Timonen P: Optimal use of cyclosporin in the treatment of Behcet's disease. Berlin: Springer-Verlag, 1988.

Behcet's Disease

Behcet's disease is a chronic, multisystem disorder characterized by recurrent episodes of uveitis, genital ulcers, oral ulcerations, and skin lesions.[1–10] The disease was initially described by Hippocrates. In this century, the disease was described by Adamantiades, a Greek ophthalmologist, and later by a Turkish dermatologist, Hulusi Behcet, in 1937. Behcet's disease is a chronic disorder characterized by an underlying vasculitis.

Epidemiology

Ocular disease has assumed great importance in certain parts of the world, such as Japan and the Middle East. Behcet's disease occurs most frequently in Japan and the Mediterranean basin. In Japan, the disease constitutes as much as 25% of all cases of uveitis, and accounts for 12% of blindness in young and middle-aged adults. The incidence and prevalence of Behcet's disease has been increasing markedly in Japan since 1959. The mean age of patients with Behcet's disease is 24 years, and the disorder occurs more frequently in men. We have observed familial occurrence of Behcet's disease which has been reported by other authors. Of 167 patients with Behcet's disease, we have found 14 patients among 6 families (unpublished data). Fam and associates[2] described a case of neonatal Behcet's, in which the mother suffered from oral and genital ulcerations and pustular cutaneous lesions. The infant was found shortly after birth to have extensive oral genital ulceration. The acute lesions resolved spontaneously in 6 weeks, leaving depressed scars. In 1972, the Behcet's Disease Research Committee of Japan established diagnostic criteria for Behcet's disease. They divided the symptoms into major and minor (Table 7.3). In the complete (definite) type, the four major criteria include ocular lesions, oral ulcers, genital ulcers, and skin lesions. In the incomplete (probable) type, ocular and one major criterion or three major criteria are observed. (Figures 7.19–7.30.)

Clinical Manifestations

Mucosal Ulcerations. Clinical features of Behcet's disease. The recurrent aphthous ulcer of the oral mucosa may occur on the lips (see Figure 7.19), gingiva, palate, and tongue. The ulcers are a diagnostic problem when they occur early in the disease. In the absence of other diagnostic criteria, it is some-

Table 7.3. Behcet's Disease

Major criteria
1. Ocular lesions
2. Aphthous ulcers
3. Genital ulcers
4. Skin lesions
Minor criteria
1. Arthritis
2. Gastroenteritis
3. Epididymitis
4. Central nervous system involvement
Complete type: All four major criteria
Incomplete type: Ocular and one major or three minor criteria

*Behcet's Disease Research Committee of Japan, 1972.

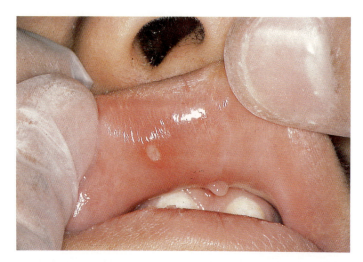

Figure 7.19. Aphthous ulcer in Behcet's disease.

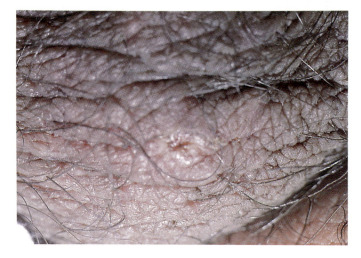

Figure 7.20. Scrotal ulceration in Behcet's disease.

times difficult to differentiate Behcet's ulcer from other recurrent aphthous ulcers. The ulcers in Behcet's disease are usually less painful than other aphthous ulcers. The aphthous ulcers of Behcet's present as localized hyperemia followed by mucosal papule, which becomes a necrotic ulcer with a gray membrane. Trauma appears to be a predisposing factor. The ulcer may heal, leaving a scar, and recurrences may occur at the same site. The lack of pain in patients with Behcet's disease may be caused by the recurrence of the ulcers at the site of scar tissue of a previous ulcer. Genital ulcers of Behcet's disease are usually painful and occur most frequently in the scrotum (see Figure 7.20) and the vulva. Ulcers heal leaving a scar, which may help to confirm the diagnosis.

Cutaneous Manifestations. Skin manifestations of Behcet's disease are common. Patients may develop erythema nodosum-like lesions, superficial thrombophlebitis, and folliculitis. Hyperirritability of the skin is also a common feature in patients with Behcet's disease. Needle puncture of the skin may lead to pustule at the site of the injection in 12 to 24 hours. This occurs in approximately 40% to 50% of the patients with Behcet's disease.

Ocular Manifestations (Table 7.4)

The most striking ocular manifestation of the disease is the anterior or posterior uveitis.[10] The eye lesions are the most serious of the major criteria and may eventuate in blindness. Table 7.4 summa-

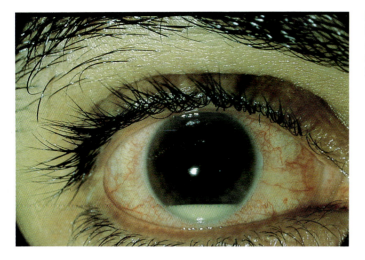

Figure 7.21. Hypopyon in a patient with Behcet's disease. (Reprinted with permission from Tabbara KF, Al Balla S: Ocular manifestations of Behcet's disease. Asia-Pacific Ophthalmol 1991;3:8–88.)

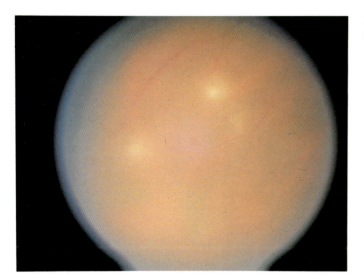

Figure 7.22. Focal areas of retinal infiltration in Behcet's disease.

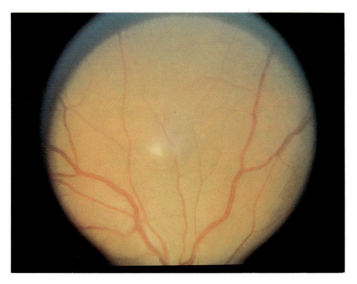

Figure 7.23. One small retinal infiltrate in Behcet's disease. Lesion resolved spontaneously.

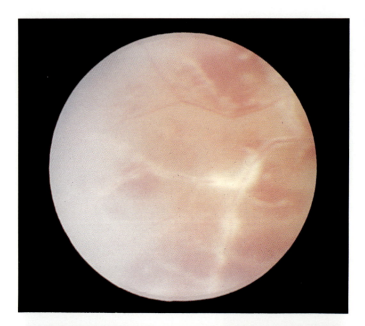

Figure 7.24. Retinal phlebitis in Behcet's disease (reprinted with permission from Tabbara KF, Al Balla S: Ocular manifestations of Behcet's disease. Asia-Pacific Ophthalmol 1991;3:8–11).

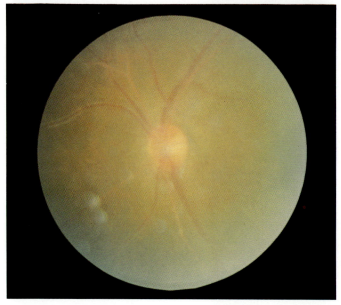

Figure 7.25. Retinal vasculitis with hyperemia of the optic nerve head.

rizes the clinical findings in patients with Behcet's disease. One of the most common characteristic findings is the presence of a sterile hypopyon (see Figure 7.21). The hypopyon may occur with severe anterior uveitis or may be seen in the absence of the inflammatory signs, a finding that we refer to as the "cold hypopyon." This may be similar to the formation of a skin pustule and may indicate a local abnormal release of chemotactic factors, which may follow local trauma. We have also observed this phenomenon, namely, the formation of

hypopyon, in patients undergoing cataract extraction. This should be kept in mind to avoid unnecessary microbiologic investigations or treatment for presumed bacterial endophthalmitis. Cataract formation, anterior and posterior synechiae, and glaucoma are common complications of the anterior uveitis in patients with Behcet's disease. Some patients may progress to phthisis bulbi, which is known as a late sequela of the disease. Glaucoma may be caused by peripheral anterior synechiae, neovascular glaucoma, or steroid-induced glau-

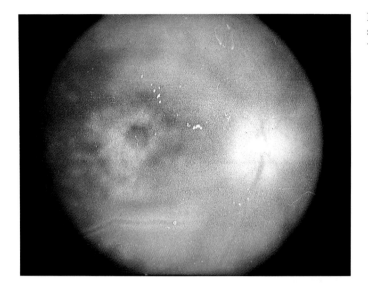

Figure 7.26. Fluorescein angiography showing evidence of leakage from a retinal vein and CME.

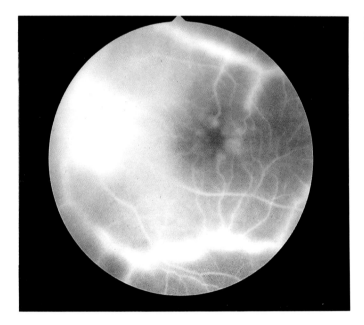

Figure 7.27. Fluorescein angiography showing retinal vascular leakage.

coma. The vitreous shows anterior vitreous cells, and the posterior segment is frequently involved in patients with Behcet's disease. The posterior manifestations of Behcet's disease include micro-vascular retinal abnormalities, retinal vasculitis, which could be phlebitis, and occasionally an ar-teritis (see Figures 7.24 and 7.25). Approximately 53% of patients with Behcet's disease develop reti-nal vasculitis.[13] The vasculitis may lead to vascular occlusion and retinal hemorrhages. Neovascular formation is seen as part of the vascular occlusive process. Focal areas of retinitis may be seen, and

cystoid macular edema may occur (Figures 7.22 and 7.23).

Fluorescein angiographic findings are character-ized by perivenous and capillary leakage (Figures 7.26 and 7.27). Leakage is seen in retinal capillar-ies in the region of the macula and optic nerve head. Perivenous leakage around the optic nerve head is also a constant feature. The precise mechanism of this endothelial disturbance is not well understood, but could be related to focal deposition of immune complexes at the basement membrane of the vascu-lar wall. Complications of Behcet's disease in the

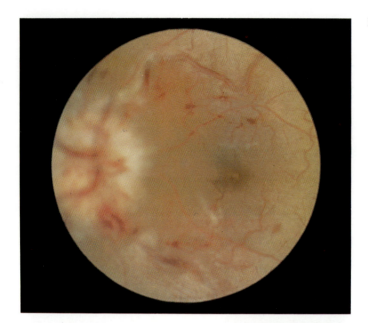

Figure 7.28. Optic papillitis and vasculitis.

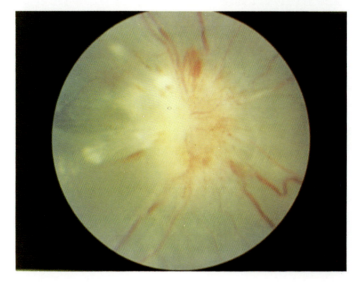

Figure 7.29. Optic nerve head edema and inflammation.

posterior segment include optic papillitis (Figures 7.28 and 7.29), and optic nerve vasculitis, which may lead to optic atrophy (Figure 7.30). Degenerative changes in the macular area may occur. Attenuation or occlusion of the retinal vessels also may occur in the late stages of disease.

Treatment

Behcet's disease is a chronic disorder with remissions and exacerbations. The objectives of therapy should be closely evaluated in each patient. The first line of therapy in this immunologically mediated disorder is corticosteroids. Whatever the short-term benefits of this therapy are, such treatment should be kept to a minimum. Several immunosuppressive agents have been used in the treatment of Behcet's disease. Table 7.5 summarizes the immunosuppressive agents that have been used in the treatment of Behcet's disease. Immunosuppressive therapy may be considered with certain guidelines in mind, as shown in Table 7.6. Chlorambucil has been advocated for patients with Behcet's disease but long-

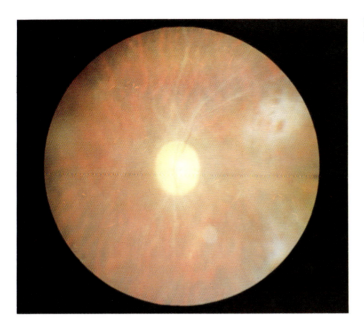

Figure 7.30. Optic atrophy in a patient with Behcet's disease.

term treatment with chlorambucil has been disappointing in some patients with this disorder.

Furthermore, chlorambucil has a harmful effect on spermatogenesis and may lead to sterility in male patients. Azathioprine at a dosage level of 150 mg orally per day in three divided doses has also been used. It seems well established that the disease results from immune derangement, and the use of agents whose action causes further immune depression defies therapeutic logic. Therapy may do little good while masking the symptoms.

Azathioprine has also been recommended for the treatment of Behcet's disease. The drug is initially given at a dosage level of 2 mg/kg/day orally with monitoring of the white blood cell count and differential. Azathioprine is given for two weeks after a clinical response is noted. It is later tapered to 1 mg/kg/day. Pulse therapy with methotrexate 7.5 mg IV weekly or every other week has also been given to patients with intractable uveitis. The long-term safety and efficacy of this regimen remains to be determined. Immunomodulators that affect T cell function such as FK 506 and cyclosporine have been used in Behcet's disease.

Clinical trials have shown that cyclosporine is effective in the treatment of patients with this disease.[11–17] The drug exerts its effect on T-cell-dependent function but has no effect on T cell response. It is believed that cyclosporine selectively inhibits the clonal proliferation of helper T cells and

may have certain inhibiting effects on chemotaxis of cyclosporine when given at a dosage of 5 mg/kg/day orally (see Chapter 12). Maintenance dose (1 to 3 mg/kg orally per day) of cyclosporine may be given for prolonged periods with no adverse effect.[15]

Mochizuki and associates evaluated the effects of FK 506 on patients with refractory uveitis.[18] Fifty-three patients (41 Behcet's, 5 Vogt-Koyanagi-Harada, 4 retinal vasculitis, and 3 other forms of uveitis) were included in this study. The authors found FK 506 given orally at a dosage of 0.10 to 0.15 mg/kg daily to be effective in suppressing the intraocular inflammation. The authors recommended to maintain the trough blood level to be between 15 and 25 ng/ml. Similar to cyclosporine, FK 506 is nephrotoxic and long-term safety and efficacy of FK 506 remains to be determined. The major adverse effects include nephrotoxicity, neurologic symptoms, gastrointestinal symptoms, and hyperglycemia. Unlike cyclosporine, FK 506 did not lead to hirsutism.

The therapeutic regimens for the treatment of autoimmune disorders have included cytotoxic, immunosuppressive, and immunomodulating agents. Autoimmune diseases have been defined and classified based on their clinical manifestations and not on their etiology. For this reason the therapy is aimed at minimizing the end-stage damage by effector immunocytes and their cytokines. The major drugs used for the treatment of noninfectious immune-me-

Table 7.4. Behcet's Disease

I. DESCRIPTION

Behcet's disease is a chronic autoimmune disorder characterized by recurrent episodes of uveitis, oral ulcerations, and skin lesions. The disease was described by Adamantiades in 1931 and Hulusi Behcet in 1937.

II. CLINICAL PRESENTATION

A. Symptoms
   1. Blurring of vision.
   2. Photophobia.
   3. Redness of the eye and sometimes patient may notice the hypopyon in the eye and complain of whitish discoloration over the iris.
   4. Other symptoms include ulcerations of the mouth and genitalia, skin rash or other skin lesions.

B. Signs
   1. Perilimbal ciliary flush.
   2. Fine keratitic precipitates.
   3. Anterior chamber cells and flare, and sometimes a sterile hypopyon is noted.
   4. Posterior synechiae.
   5. Complicated cataract.

C. Posterior Signs
   1. Vitreous cells, strands or opacities.
   2. Retinal vasculitis (phlebitis or arthritis).
   3. Retinal hemorrhages.
   4. Retinal neovascularization.
   5. Focal retinitis.
   6. Papillitis and peripapillary flame-shape hemorrhages with retinal edema.
   7. Cystoid macular edema.

D. Types of Behcet's Disease
   Two types are identified:
   1. Definite Behcet's (complete type): All four major criteria of the disease are observed (ocular lesions, skin lesions, genital ulcers, and oral ulcers).

Table 7.4. (continued)

   2. Probable Behcet's (incomplete type): Ocular lesion with one other major criterion or three minor criteria.

E. Major Criteria of Behcet's Disease
   1. Ocular lesions.
   2. Skin lesions.
   3. Genital ulcers.
   4. Oral ulcers.

F. Minor Criteria of Behcet's Disease
   1. Arthritis.
   2. Gastroenteritis.
   3. Eipdidymitis.
   4. Central nervous system involvement.
   5. Others.
   Behcet's disease is characterized by remissions and exacerbations with variable course and outcome.

III. LABORATORY TESTS

A. Pathergy skin tests. Skin puncture with a needle may cause the formation of a pustule within 12 to 24 hours after the puncture.
B. Complete blood counts and urinalysis.
C. Serum immune complexes may be elevated.
D. HLA typing. Patients with Behcet's disease have an association with HLA B51.
E. Elevated immunoglobulins may be demonstrated in some patients during the activity of the disease.

IV. TREATMENT

A. Oral corticosteroids.
B. Colchicine.
C. Immunosuppressive therapy, chlorambucil or azathioprine.
D. Cyclosporine in patients with active vasculitis or severe papillitis.
E. Thalidomide may be helpful in patients with erythema nodosum and in oral and genital ulcerations. (Thalidomide is a teratogenic agent.)
F. Investigational: Oral feeding of retinal S-antigen.

diated uveitis include: corticosteriods, alkylating agents (cyclophosphamide and chlorambucil), antimetabolites (azathioprine and methotrexate), and immunomodulators such as cyclosporine and FK 506. All these agents have been used for the treatment of Behcet's disease either simply or in combination. Despite advances in the field of immunology, genetics, molecular biology, and pharmacology, autoimmune diseases including Behcet's disease remain diseases of unknown etiology that have no definitive cure.

Tabbara and Chavis studied retrospectively the long-term visual outcome of patients with complete Behcet's disease.[19] The authors compared the visual outcome of patients on cyclosporine and prednisone to those who received conventional therapy in the form of chlorambucil or azathioprine. A total of 63 patients with complete Behcet's disease were included. All patients had retinal vasculitis at the time of presentation. There were 60 men and 3 women. Thirty-five patients received cyclosporine 5 mg/kg/day orally and prednisone 1 mg/kg/day orally, and 28 patients received conventional therapy consisting of oral chlorambucil 0.1 mg/kg/day or oral azathioprine 2 mg/kg/day. Patients were given treatment during the active phases of the disease and treatment was tapered two weeks after a therapeutic response was noted and was to be discontinued

Table 7.5. Immunosuppressive Agents Used in Behcet's Disease and Other Forms of Immune-Mediated Uveitis

Drug	Initial Dose (oral unless otherwise indicated)	Major Adverse Effects
Prednisone	1 mg/kg/day	Obesity, electrolyte disbalance, osteoporosis
Cyclophosphamide	2 mg/kg/day	Leukopenia, cystitis
Chlorambucil	0.1 mg/kg/day	Leukopenia, thrombocytopenia, azospermia
Azathioprine	2 mg/kg/day	Leukopenia, thrombocytopenia, azospermia
Methotrexate	7.5 mg IV once every other week	Leukopenia, thrombocytopenia
Cyclosporine	5 mg/kg/day (maintenance dose 1 to 3 mg/kg/day)	Nephrotoxicity, hepatotoxicity, hirsutism, neurologic symptoms, GI symptoms
FK 506	0.15 mg/kg/day	Similar to Cyclosporine except for hirsutism

Table 7.6. Guidelines for the Use of Immunosuppressive Therapy

1. Reversible, vision-threatening lesions must be present.
2. The condition must not respond to conventional therapy.
3. There must be meticulous follow-up study: complete blood count, platelet counts, and sperm counts in male patients.
4. There must be an objective evaluation of ocular findings.
5. The course of treatment should be short (not to exceed 6 weeks).
6. The total cumulative dose of chlorambucil should not exceed 8.2 mg/kg per course of treatment.
7. There must be no active infection and no hematologic contraindication.
8. The therapy should have the patient's informed consent.

when intraocular inflammatory signs had subsided. Patients were followed up for a period of 20 to 124 months with a mean follow-up period of 61 months.

At a mean follow-up period of 60 months, 8 (23%) patients out of 35 patients on intermittent oral cyclosporine had a visual acuity of 20/50 or better. On the other hand, 7 (25%) out of 28 patients on conventional immunosuppressive therapy had a visual acuity of 20/50 or better. Three patients had developed phthisis bulbi (one on cyclosporine and two on conventional therapy with chlorambucil or azathioprine). Three patients underwent enucleation of one eye.

Seven patients had no light perception in one eye (3 in the cyclosporine and 4 in the conventional therapy group). One out of five patients was blind in each treatment group and 30 (48%) out of 63 patient were blind in one eye after treatment. There was no statistically significant difference in the visual outcome between patients on cyclosporine and those on chlorambucil or azathioprine.[19]

This study has demonstrated that the current recommended therapeutic regimens of cyclosporine or other conventional immunosuppressive therapy (chlorambucil or azathioprine) are inadequate for the control or amelioration of chronic uveitis in pa-

tients with severe Behcet's disease. Therapy did not prevent the loss of vision. It is recognized that short-term therapy of patients with Behcet's disease may lead to suppression of the intraocular inflammation. Persistent subclinical inflammation and vasculitis may lead to structural damage of the ocular structures. Behcet's disease is a chronic disorder that may lead to intraocular inflammation that may be mild or severe. The disease is also characterized by spontaneous remissions and exacerbations. The question of whether we are modifying the final visual outcome in Behcet's disease remains to be determined.

The ocular tissue bioavailability was assessed in pigmented and albino rabbits.[20] Cyclosporine tissue levels by a specific monoclonal antibody radioimmunoassay. Cyclosporine levels in the iris and retina-choroid were significantly higher ($p < 0.01$) in the pigmented rabbits than in the albino rabbits.[20] It is of great therapeutic interest to know that cyclosporine concentrates in the uvea, the target tissue of treatment in patients with uveitis. This phenomenon may have important clinical implications. In view of the cyclosporine nephrotoxicity, lower doses of oral cyclosporine may be justified because of its high uptake and concentration in the uveal tissue. The drugs, therefore, may be given at a low dose, 1 to 3 mg/kg/day orally, and stays effective without nephrotoxicity.

Studies on oral feeding of retinal S antigen in the treatment of Behcet's disease are underway at the National Institutes of Health. The administration of oral retinal S antigen in patients who show positive serum antibody response to retinal S antigen may induce tolerance (see the Appendix).

References

1. Tabbara KF: Chlorambucil in Behcet's disease: A reappraisal. Ophthalmology 1983;90:906.
2. Fam AG, Siminovitch KA, Carette S: Neonatal Behcet's syndrome in an infant of a mother with the disease. Ann Rheum Dis 1981;40:509.
3. Lehner T, Almeida JD, Lenvisky RJ: Damaged membrane fragments and immune complexes in the blood of patients with Behcet's syndrome. Clin Exp Immunol 1978;34:206.
4. Levinsky RJ, Lehner T: Circulating soluble immune complexes in recurrent oral ulceration and Behcet's syndrome. Clin Exp Immunol 1978;32:193.
5. Editorial: Behcet's disease. Jpn J Ophthalmol 1974; 18:291.
6. Chamberlain MA: A family study of Behcet's syndrome. Ann Rheum Dis 1978;37:459.
7. Sobel JD, Haim S, Obedeanu T, et al.: Polymorphonuclear leukocyte function in Behcet's disease. J Clin Pathol 1977;30:250–253.
8. Ehrlich GE: Phagocytes and mediations of inflammation in Behcet's syndrome. International Conference on Behcet's Disease, October 1981, Tokyo, Japan.
9. Nussenblatt RB, Palestine AG, Chan CC: Cyclosporine: A therapy in the treatment of intraocular inflammatory disease resistant to systemic corticosteroids and cytotoxic agents. Am J Ophthalmol 1983;96:275–282.
10. Tabbara KF, Al Balla S: Ocular manifestations of Behcet's disease. Asia-Pacific Ophthalmol 1991;3:8–11.
11. Laupacis AMD, Keown PA, Ulan RA, et al.: Cyclosporine A: A powerful immunosuppressant. Can Med Assoc J 1982;126:1041–1046.
12. DeVries J, Baarsma GS, Zaal MJW, et al.: Cyclosporine in the treatment of severe chronic idiopathis uveitis. Br J Ophthalmol 1990;74:344–349.
13. Chavis PS, Tabbara KF: Cyclosporine in noninfectious posterior uveitis. In Recent Advances in Uveitis. Dernouchamps JP, Verougstraete C, Caspers-Velu L, Tassignon MJ (eds.). Amsterdam, The Netherlands: Kugler Publications, 1993, pp. 509–511.
14. Chavis PS, Antonios SR, Tabbara KF: Cyclosporine effects on optic nerve and retinal vasculitis in Behcet's disease. Documenta Ophthalmologica 1992;80: 133–142.
15. Whitcup SM, Salvo EC, Nussenblatt RB: Combined cyclosporine and corticosteroid therapy for sight-threatening uveitis in Behcet's disease. Am J Ophthalmol 1994;118:39–45.
16. Diaz-Llopis M, Cervera M, Menezo JL: Cyclosporin A treatment of Behcet's disease. A long-term study. Curr Eye Res 1990;9 (Suppl):17.
17. Nussenblatt RB, Palestine AG, Chan CC, et al.: Randomized, double-masked study of cyclosporine compared to prednisolone in the treatment of endogenous uveitis. Am J Ophthalmol 1991;112:138–146.
18. Mochizuki M, Masuda K, Sakane T, et al.: A clinical trial of FK 506 in refractory uveitis. Am J Ophthalmol 1993;115:763–769.
19. Tabbara KF, Chavis PS: Long-term visual outcome in patients with Behcet's disease. Proceedings of the Sixth International Symposium of the Immunology and Immunopathology of the Eye, Bethesda, Maryland, June 22–24, 1994, Elsevier Science Publishers.
20. Tabbara KF, El-Sayed YM, Cooper H, Nowailaty S: Ocular bioavailability of cyclosporine in pigmented and albino rabbits. In Recent Advances in Uveitis. Dernouchamps JP, Verougstraete C, Caspers-Velu L, Tassignon MJ (eds.). Amsterdam, The Netherlands: Kugler Publications, 1993, pp. 501–507.

Chapter 8
Other Disorders

Khalid F. Tabbara

Sarcoidosis

Ocular involvement of sarcoidosis is a common manifestation of a generalized disease. The uveal tract is frequently involved during the course of a systemic granulomatous disease. Sarcoidosis is a disease of undetermined origin, and the exact pathogenesis is not well understood.[1-7] The ocular lesions may sometimes precede or occur independently of the pulmonary sarcoidosis. Sarcoidosis has a worldwide distribution with an incidence ranging between 1 and 8 per 10,000. It is estimated that approximately 7% of all forms of sarcoidosis are associated with ocular signs.

Clinical Findings

Ocular involvement with sarcoidosis may involve any ocular structure and may involve the adnexa. Lid granulomas may occur along with conjunctival granulomas. The orbit and lacrimal glands may be involved. The cornea may show evidence of interstitial keratitis with peripheral inferior involvement causing peripheral thickening of the cornea (Figure 8.1). Sarcoid uveitis usually appears as a chronic insidious disease. There is often blurring of vision, and patients may complain of floaters. Occasionally patients may present with acute onset of pain and photophobia. Secondary glaucoma may complicate the course of anterior granulomatous uveitis. Posterior synechiae may occur and iris nodules, either Bussacca or Koeppe nodules, may develop. Anterior vitreous snowballs may occur.

Synechiae formation is common in sarcoidosis, particularly at the site of Koeppe nodule formation. Complicated cataract is also common. Extensive exudation of the vitreous may occur; the cornea may show large keratitic precipitates.

The retina is commonly involved in sarcoidosis with perivasculitis and phlebitis (Figure 8.2). Perivascular sheathing of the retinal blood vessels is common. In addition, patients may show evidence of the characteristic candle wax drippings associated with localized phlebitis. Obliteration of the retinal vessels may lead to neovascularization. Optic nerve granulomas may occur.

Histopathologically, sarcoid nodules and granulomas show epithelioid cells and giant cells characteristic of noncaseating granuloma (Figures 8.3 and 8.4). In the granuloma there is marked increase in the T-suppressor lymphocytes. Polyclonal B lymphocyte activation is characteristic of this disease. It may suggest a defect in collaboration between B lymphocyte and the activated phagocytes. Several immunologic abnormalities have been reported in this disease. Histopathologic evaluation of the granuloma in sarcoidosis shows evidence of epithelioid cells and giant cells. The granuloma is typically noncaseating.

Laboratory Diagnosis

Chest radiograph of patients with ocular sarcoidosis may show evidence of bilateral hilar adenopathy. A normal chest radiograph, however, does not rule out ocular sarcoidosis.

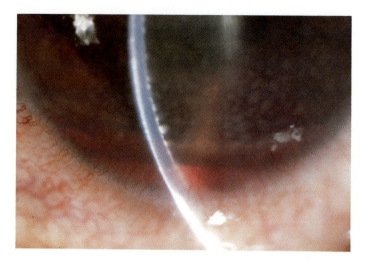

Figure 8.1. Inferior corneal thickening in a patient with sarcoidosis.

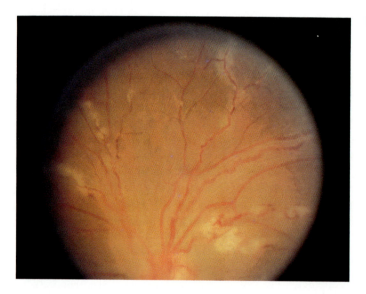

Figure 8.2. Retinal vasculitis in sarcoidosis.

Serum lysozyme is found to be elevated in sarcoidosis, but the test is not specific for this disease. Serum lysozyme may also be increased in patients with tuberculosis, Crohn's disease, and leprosy. There appears to be a high correlation between the serum lysozyme level and the activity of sarcoidosis. Serum angiotensin-converting enzyme (ACE) level may be found to be elevated in leprosy and Gaucher disease. The source of the ACE is probably the giant cells. Furthermore, there appears to be a high correlation between the serum ACE level and the activity as well as the extent of sarcoidosis. Tear levels of lysozyme and ACE may be found to be elevated in ocular sarcoidosis, but the serum levels are not. Another laboratory diagnostic test for sar-

coidosis includes the presence of cutaneous energy. It should be emphasized that a positive PPD may be present in some patients with sarcoidosis. Calcium level in the blood may be elevated if there is bony involvement. Serum protein alteration may occur, and gallium scanning is useful for assessing the presence of specific infiltration of the lacrimal and salivary glands as well as the presence of visceral lymphadenopathy.

Approximately 90% of all sarcoid patients show negative results from inoculation of skin test of antigens intradermally. The skin tests that are commonly used include *Candida,* mumps, trichophyton, and streptokinase–streptodornase antigens. The skin test indicates a decrease in the cell-

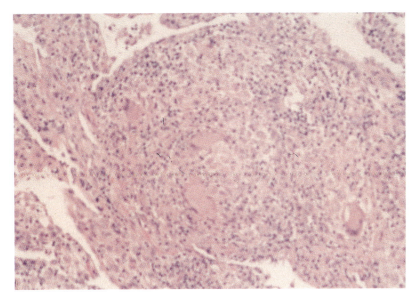

Figure 8.3. Noncaseating granuloma in sarcoidosis (100×).

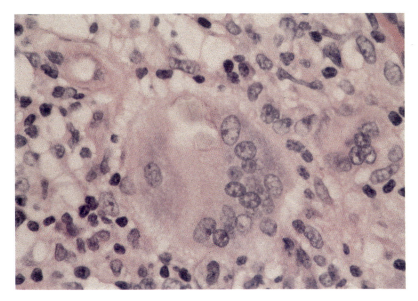

Figure 8.4. Giant cell in a conjunctival sarcoid granuloma (400×).

mediated immunity and deficiency of the T-cell interaction. Serum protein analysis may show evidence of excessive immunoglobulin production. The most significant elevation being in the gamma G immunoglobulin (IgG) fraction. Obtaining a biopsy specimen of a sarcoid nodule in the conjunctiva may show the typical noncaseating granuloma of sarcoidosis. Such biopsy specimen are generally rewarding only when there is evidence of conjunctival infiltration. The Kveim test, which requires subcutaneous injection of extracts of human sarcoid suspects, has been abandoned.

Treatment

The treatment of ocular sarcoidosis includes the use of topical, periocular, and systemic administration of corticosteroids. Initial therapy consists of prednisone 1 mg/kg/day orally. The treatment is tapered two weeks after a therapeutic response is noted. Topical application of cycloplegia and mydriasis is necessary to prevent synechiae formation. Secondary glaucoma may develop in some patients with application of antiglaucomatous therapy such as timolol maleate 0.5% eyedrops twice daily or dipivefrin 1% eyedrops twice daily. Systemic therapy with cyclosporine has been recommended. Patients may be given low-dose cyclosporine 1 to 3 mg/kg/day orally.

Geographic Choroiditis (Serpiginous Choroiditis)

Geographic choroiditis is also referred to as serpiginous choroiditis or helicoid choroidopathy. This affects all races, and patients in the age groups of 40 to 60 years appear to be more susceptible than others. The disease is a form of recurrent choroiditis of unknown cause.

Clinical Findings

Patients with geographic choroiditis present with history of blurring of vision. On examination, the anterior chamber is clear in most patients. The vitreous reaction may be variable with minimal or no inflammatory cells. The posterior segment may show a snakelike progressive choroiditis in the peripapillary region thus the term serpiginous. The active advancing edge of the helicoid choroidopathy keeps pace with the healing and the lesion may reach the macular area. When the macular is involved, vision is reduced. In most patients with geographic choroiditis, involvement of the peripapillary area leaves an atrophic choroid but may not lead to decrease in vision.

Laboratory Diagnosis

The diagnosis of geographic choroiditis is made by clinical findings and by fluorescein angiography and by ruling out other causes of choroiditis. The clinical lesions are typical, and the fluorescein angiography documents the presence of early blockage and late leakage of the dye.

Treatment

Oral corticosteroids are not effective in this disease. Pulse therapy with 500 to 1,000 mg methylprednisolone may be helpful in cases with obvious clinical signs of inflammation. Oral low-dose cyclosporine may induce remissions and prevent progression of the disease.[8] The use of azathioprine, cyclosporine, and prednisone in combination may induce rapid remission of active serpiginous choroiditis.[9] The disease may recur immediately after therapy is discontinued.[8,9] This may indicate the need for placing some patients with active serpiginous choroiditis on a maintenance regimen. The dosage recommended for the triple therapy includes cyclosporine 5 mg/kg/day, azathioprine 1.5 mg/kg/day, and prednisone 1 mg/kg/day orally for two weeks after a therapeutic response is noted. Following this regimen, prednisone is tapered to 0.5 mg/kg/day for two weeks and then switched to alternate-day therapy. Azathioprine and cyclosporine are tapered over the next four weeks. Maintenance therapy consists of prednisone 0.5 mg/kg/day orally every other day and cyclosporine 2 to 3 mg/kg/day orally.

References

1. Boeck C: Multipelt benignt hud-sarkoid. Norsk Mag laegevidensk 1899;1321–1334.
2. James DG. Ocular sarcoidosis. Ann NY Acad Sci 1986:465;551–563.
3. Baarsma GS, La Hey E, Glasius E, et al.: The predictive value of serum angiotensin converting enzyme and lysozyme levels in the diagnosis of ocular sarcoidosis. Am J Ophthalmol 1987;104:211–217.
4. Weinreb RN, Tessler H: Laboratory diagnosis of ophthalmic sarcoidosis. Surv Ophthalmol 1984;28:653–664.
5. Palestine AG, Nussenblatt RB, Chan CC: Treatment of intraocular complications of sarcoidosis. Ann NY Acad Sci 1986;465:564–574.
6. Brod RD: Presumed sarcoid choroidopathy mimicking birdshot retinochoroidopathy. Am J Ophthamol 1990; 109(3):357–358.
7. Karma A, Huhti E, Poukkula A: Course and outcome of ocular sarcoidosis. Am J Ophthalmol 1988;106:467–472.
8. Secchi AG, Tognon MS, Moro F: Cyclosporine-A in the treatment of serpiginous choroiditis. In Belfort R, Jr., Petrelli AMN, Nussenblatt R (eds.). World Uveitis Symposium: Proceedings of the First World Uveitis Symposium held in Guarujá, Sao Paulo 63 Brazil, 1988. Sao Paulo: Livraria Roca, 1989; 631–636.
9. Hooper PL, Kaplan HJ: Triple agent immunosuppression in serpiginous choroiditis. Ophthalmology 1991;98: 944–952.

Chapter 9
Tumor-Induced Posterior Uveitis

Khalid F. Tabbara

Several types of intraocular tumors may cause intraocular inflammatory diseases (Figures 9.1 to 9.11). Malignant melanoma of the choroid and retinoblastoma of the retina are two examples. Inflammatory reactions in such lesions may be caused by necrosis within the tumor or may be secondary to immunologically mediated reaction to the tumor cell surface antigens. We have seen patients with ciliary body malignant melanoma presented as chronic panuveitis. Such intraocular tumors, therefore, should be considered in the differential diagnosis of posterior uveitis and intermediate uveitis. Hematologic and lymphoproliferative disorders, however, may infiltrate the choroid, leading to a diffuse form of choroiditis (Figure 9.6 to 9.8). This may occur in acute myelogenous and promonocytic leukemia, as well as in several other types of lymphoproliferative disorders (Figures 9.9 and 9.11). One entity, primary clear cell or CNS lymphoma (reticulum cell sarcoma) of the retina, may masquerade as uveitis.

Reticulum Cell Sarcoma (CNS Lymphoma)

The term *reticulum cell sarcoma* is a misnomer. This is not a true type of sarcoma but rather central nervous system (CNS) lymphoma. This is a B-cell lymphoma. Primary lymphoma of the retina is very rare and occurs in the older age group. In most cases the intraocular lymphoma of the retina precedes or complicates an intracerebral manifestation of malignant lymphoma. The lesion appears as a retinal creamy-white lesion with sharp borders and evidence of cells in the vitreous. The disease presents with a lymphomatous infiltration of the subretinal pigment epithelial space and vitreous and can masquerade as chronic uveitis in elderly patients.

The predominant symptom consists of seeing floaters and a decrease in vision associated with headaches and neurologic deterioration.

Patients develop anterior mild uveitis with fine keratitic precipitates. Cells in the vitreous are seen, and the lesions in the posterior segment appear as yellowish multiple subretinal pigment epithelial infiltration. The lesion also may infiltrate the choroid. Hyperemia of the optic nerve head may occur. The disease is bilateral in 80% of the cases.

Laboratory Diagnosis

The diagnosis of CNS lymphoma of the retina requires obtaining a vitreous biopsy specimen, which then is subjected to cytospin and cytologic examination. Lumbar puncture may demonstrate neoplastic cells in the cerebrospinal fluid. Magnetic resonance imaging or computerized tomography (CT) scan may show evidence of CNS involvement.

Treatment

Treatment of CNS lymphoma is part of the treatment of the CNS lymphocytic infiltration. Prophylactic irradiation of the eye and prophylactic irradiation of the brain may be indicated. Vitrectomy may induce visual rehabilitation in patients who have evidence of vitreous infiltration. Chemotherapy consisting of

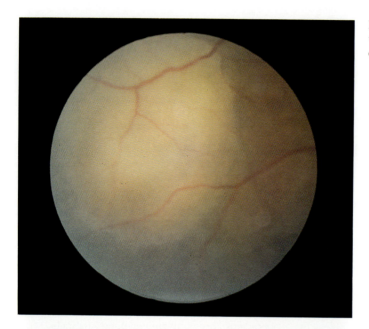

Figure 9.1. A posterior segment lesion involving the choroid. Patient had carcinoma of the breast with metastasis to the eye.

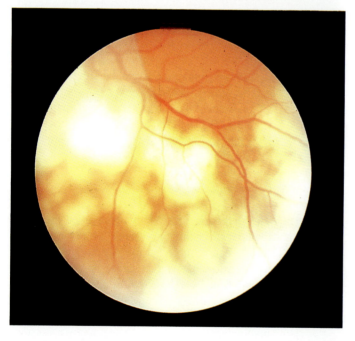

Figure 9.2. Reticulum cell sarcoma (CNS lymphoma or giant cell lymphoma).

IV methotrexate may be helpful. The treatment may have to be repeated in cycles with leucovivin rescue.

Leukemia

Human T-cell lymphotropic virus type I is a retrovirus that has worldwide distribution. The virus causes infection in humans.[1] HTLV-I endemic areas include Southwest Japan, Central Africa, and the Caribbean Islands.[2] The disease is transmitted by blood transfusions, sexual contacts, and breast feeding. The virus has been identified as a cause of adult T-cell leukemia. Patients may develop myelopathy[1] and the disease progresses rapidly. Myelopathy associated with HTLV-I is common. Patients develop weakness and spasticity of the lower extremities, bowel dysfunction, back pain,

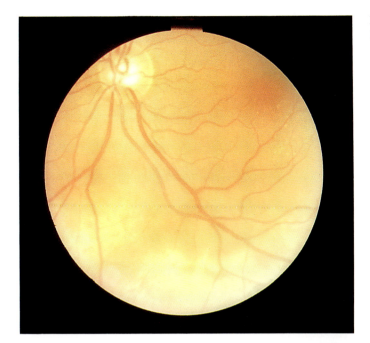

Figure 9.3. Reticulum cell sarcoma (CNS lymphoma) in a 65-year-old man.

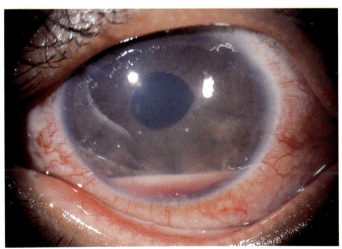

Figure 9.4. Pseudohypopyon in a patient with non-Hodgkin's lymphoma.

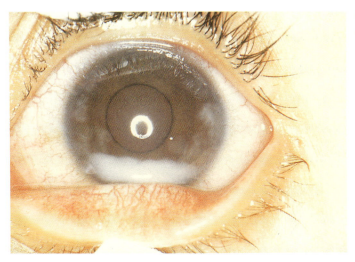

Figure 9.5. Mashed-potato–like pseudohypopyon in a patient with retinoblastoma.

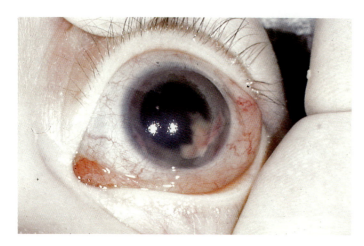

Figure 9.6. Eight-month-old infant with promonocytic leukemia and pseudohypopyon. Patient had choroidal involvement, as shown in Figures 9.7 and 9.8.

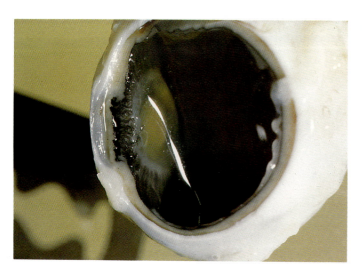

Figure 9.7. Diffuse choroidal thickening secondary to leukemia infiltration.

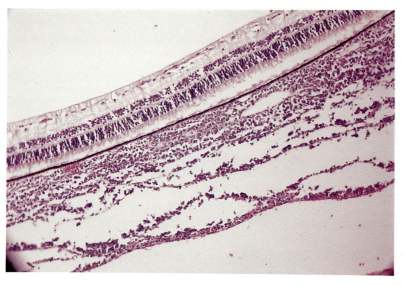

Figure 9.8. Histopathologic H & E–stained section (100×) showing choroidal infiltration by leukemia cells in the periphery. The retina was not involved.

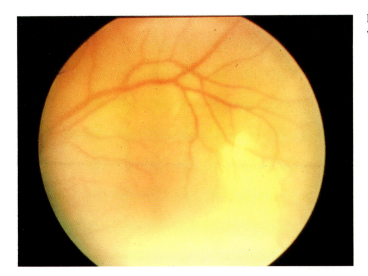

Figure 9.9. Non-Hodgkin's lymphoma with posterior segment involvement.

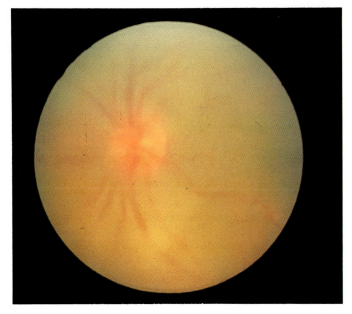

Figure 9.10. Posterior uveitis in a patient with Hodgkin's disease.

and neurological symptoms. Ocular findings consist of retinal vasculitis,[3] cotton-wool spots, cytomegalovirus retinitis, and uveitis.[4] Vitreous exudates and snowball-like opacities may be seen.[4] Vitrectomy specimens have shown that the snowballs were leukemic cells.

Patients may develop deep retinal and subretinal infiltrates without vitreous exudates.[5] A chorioretinal biopsy specimen of these retinal infiltrates revealed a large number of atypical mononuclear cells at the level of the retinal pigment epithelium.[5] Electron microscopy showed cellular features consistent with T-cell lymphoma/leukemia.[5] HTLV-I can be verified by polymerase chain reaction conducted on peripheral blood mononuclear cells.[5,6] Mochizuki and co-workers reported a significant association between HTLV-I infection and uveitis.[6] The patients were in the third and fourth decade and had an intermediate uveitis characterized by mild to moderate involvement of the vitreous. Patients had retinal vasculitis and iritis.[6] The differential diagnosis should include other causes of uveitis, intermediate uveitis, Vogt-Koyanagi-Harada, and sarcoidosis.

Proviral DNA of human T-cell lymphotropic virus type I can be detected by polyermase chain reaction by using pol region primers from the

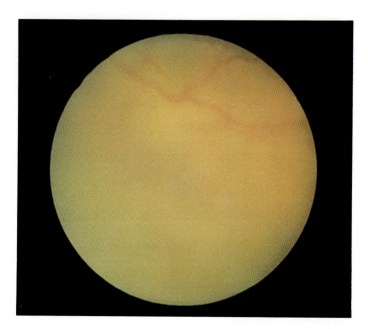

Figure 9.11. Peripheral retina of same patient shown in Figure 9.10.

inflammatory cells in the anterior chamber.[6] Intermediate uveitis appears to be an important manifestation of HTLV-I infection. HTLV-I infection, therefore, should be ruled out in patients presenting with intermediate uveitis and retinal vasculitis in edemic areas.

Ocular Leukemia

The ocular structures are frequently the site of leukemic infiltration. All types of leukemia may involve the eye. The most common site of leukemic cellular infiltrates is the choroid. Leukemic cells may cause iritis, iridocyclitis, secondary glaucoma, and vitritis. This masquerade syndrome is important to diagnose. The eye symptoms could be the presenting clinical manifestation of leukemia.[7] Patients may develop severe anterior uveitis and hypopyon.

In patients with non-Hodgkins lymphoma, the anterior segment is more frequently affected and they may present with iritis and hypopyon.

Metastatic Lesions

Metastatic lesions of the eye may complicate the course of several types of systemic malignancies, including carcinoma of the breast (Figure 9.1), carcinoma of the lung, or carcinoma of the prostate.

Metastatic lesions may lead to focal, yellowish elevated lesions in the subretinal space, giving the appearance of peau d'orange.

References

1. Osame M, Usuku K, Izumo S, et al.: HTLV-I associated myelopathy, a new clinical entity. Lancet 1986;1: 1031–1032.
2. Blattner WA: Epidemiology of HTLV-I and associated diseases. In Blattner WA (ed.). Human Retrovirology: HTLV. New York, NY: Raven Press; 1990:251–265.
3. Hayasaka S, Takatori Y, Noda S, et al.: Retinal vasculitis in a mother and her son with human T-lymphotropic virus type 1 associated myelopathy. Br J Ophthalmol 1991;75:566–567.
4. Ohba N, Matsumoto M, Sameshima M, et al.: Ocular manifestations in patients infected with human T-lymphotropic virus type I. Jpn J Ophthalmol 1989;33:1–12.
5. Kumar SR, Gill PS, Wagner DG, et al.: Human T-cell lymphotropic virus type-I associated retinal lymphoma. Arch Ophthalmol 1994;112:954–959.
6. Mochizuki M, Watanabe T, Yamaguchi K, et al.: Uveitis associated with human T-cell lymphotropic virus type I. Am J Ophthamol 1992;114:123–129.
7. Tabbara KF, Beckstead JJ: Acute promonocytic leukemia with ocular involvement. Arch Ophthalmol 1980;98: 1055–1058.

Chapter 10
Differential Diagnosis of Posterior Uveitis

Khalid F. Tabbara

The term *posterior uveitis* has been used to denote inflammatory processes of both the retina and choroid. Both the retina and choroid are targets of a variety of immunologic, infectious, and malignant disorders. Such inflammations are common, and one rarely sees a disease affecting the retina or choroid without having a spillover to the other tissue. The retina and the choroid, however, may be selectively afflicted by various autoimmune disorders or infectious agents. Such inflammations may start either in the retina or the choroid. Based on the basic immunopathogenesis of the tissue involved (e.g., vasculitis in Behcet's disease), and the biologic characteristics of the infectious agent, the retina, choroid, or both may be affected. The diagnosis of posterior uveitis can be established on the basis of (1) the medical history, including racial background, geographic location of the patient, personal habits, the symptoms, and mode of onset of the disease; (2) the clinical findings; (3) the association with a systemic disease; and (4) the laboratory findings.

This chapter discusses the differential diagnosis of posterior uveitis and elucidates the clinical signs and symptoms that differentiates one entity from the other (Figures 10.1 through 10.15).

Causes of Posterior Uveitis

There are several systemic and ocular diseases that may lead to posterior uveitis.[1-8] Table 10.1 demonstrates the various disorders that might afflict the posterior segment of the eye, leading to posterior uveitis. Certain clinical manifestations of posterior uveitis may suggest the nature of the diagnostic entity and point to the diagnosis. To make sense out of a confusing subject, one has to retrieve the facts and dissect the clinical observation in a systematic manner, narrowing the differential diagnosis to a short list, focusing on entities that may lead to the disease entity based on history and clinical observation. The laboratory tests are used only to refine the clinical diagnosis and to rule out certain entities. The prevalence of various causes of posterior uveitis may vary from one geographic location to another, from one country to another, and sometimes within regions of the same country.

In a patient with posterior uveitis, the age, sex, geographic location, and race of patient, as well as the history, mode of onset, and laterality of the condition, should be considered. The signs and symptoms of the presenting disorder should be recorded. From the point of view of morphology, the lesions in the posterior segment can be focal, geographic, or diffuse. Those that cause clouding of the overlying vitreous should be differentiated from those that never cause vitreous cells. In addition, the lesions that are regularly associated with retinal vasculitis or with serous detachment of the retina must be separately designated. The type and distribution of the vitreous opacities also must be stipulated. Inflammatory lesions of the posterior segment are generally insidious in their onset, but some may be accompanied by the abrupt development of vitreous clouding and visual loss. As a general rule, such diseases are accompanied by anterior uveitis, which in turn is sometimes associated with a form of secondary glaucoma.

Table 10.1. Causes of Posterior Uveitis

I. INFECTIOUS DISORDERS
    A. Viruses: CMV, herpes simplex, herpes zoster, rubella, rubeola, human immune deficiency virus, Epstein–Barr virus, Coxsackie virus. Probable viral cause: acute retinal necrosis.
    B. Bacteria: *Mycobacterium tuberculosis,* brucellosis, sporadic and endemic syphilis, *Nocardia, Neisseria meningitis, Mycobacterium avium,* Yersinia, and Borrelia (cause of Lyme disease).
    C. Fungi: *Candida, Histoplasma, Cryptococcus, Aspergillus.*
    D. Parasites: *Toxoplasma, Toxocara, Cysticercus,* and *Onchocerca.*

II. NONINFECTIOUS DISORDERS
    A. Autoimmune
        1. Behcet's
        2. Vogt-Koyanagi-Harada
        3. Periarteritis nodosa
        4. Sympathetic ophthalmia
        5. Retinal vasculitis
    B. Malignancy
        1. Reticulum cell sarcoma
        2. Leukemia
        3. Metastatic lesions
    C. UNKNOWN CAUSE
        1. Sarcoidosis
        2. Geographic choroiditis
        3. Acute multifocal placoid pigment epitheliopathy
        4. Birdshot retinopathy
        5. Retinal pigment epitheliopathy (Hepatitis C)

Age in the Differential Diagnosis of Posterior Uveitis

Posterior uveitis seen in patients between birth and 3 years of age may be caused by retinoblastoma or leukemia. Autoimmune disorders are rare in this age group, whereas infectious diseases of the posterior pole may include congenitally acquired infections such as cytomegalovirus (CMV) disease, toxoplasmosis, syphilis, herpetic retinitis, and rubella infection.

In the age group of 4 to 15 years, the causes of posterior uveitis may include toxocariasis, toxoplasmosis, intermediate uveitis, CMV, masquerade syndrome, and subacute sclerosing panencephalitis. Autoimmune diseases such as sympathetic ophthalmia may occur in this age group, and the course may be severe and fulminant. Other autoimmune diseases such as Vogt-Koyanagi-Harada syndrome, Behcet's disease, and vasculitis may occur in this age group. Sarcoidosis rarely has its onset in this age group.

In the age group of 16 to 40 years the differential diagnosis of posterior uveitis includes sarcoidosis, sympathetic ophthalmia, Behcet's disease, Vogt-Koyanagi-Harada syndrome, toxoplasmosis, Lyme disease, and, less frequently, endogenous bacterial or fungal infections. In this age group acquired immune deficiency syndrome (AIDS) may occur more frequently than in other age groups, and endogenous opportunistic infections of the retina and choroid are common. Patients who present with posterior

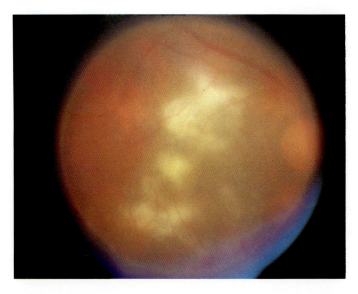

Figure 10.1. A 60-year old man with tuberculous chorioretinitis. Patient responded to systemic antituberculous therapy.

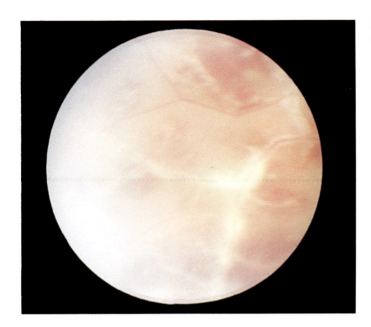

Figure 10.2. Retinal vasculitis (phlebitis) in a patient with Behcet's disease.

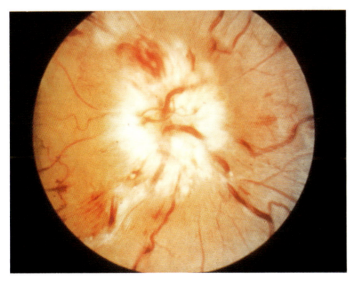

Figure 10.3. Optic papillitis and retinal vasculitis in a patient with Behcet's disease.

uveitis and are older than 40 years of age may have endogenous viral, bacterial, fungal, or parasitic infections (e.g., herpes ARN, CMV retinitis, Lyme tuberculosis, cryptococcosis, toxoplasmosis) or CNS lymphoma. Autoimmune diseases are rare in this age group.

Sex, Race, Geographic Location

Certain autoimmune disorders causing posterior uveitis are more common in men, for example, Behcet's disease, whereas others show no sex

predilection, for example, Vogt-Koyanagi-Harada syndrome and sympathetic ophthalmia. Women are more commonly affected with systemic lupus erythematosus.

Sarcoidosis is more common in blacks living in the United States and rare among blacks living in South Africa or other countries such as Saudi Arabia. Behcet's disease is common in Japan and the Mediterranean basin. Toxoplasmosis is a common cause of posterior uveitis in many western countries and South America and rare in Alaska and Siberia.

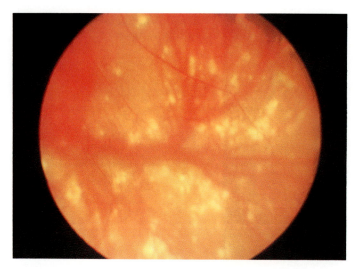

Figure 10.4. Fundus photo of a 15-year-old male patient with sympathetic ophthalmia. Note multiple Dalen-Fuchs nodules.

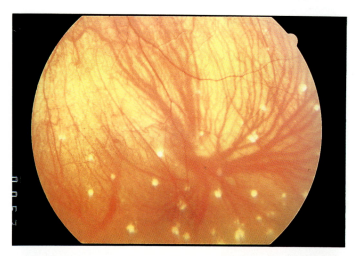

Figure 10.5. Fundus photo of a 19-year-old woman with Vogt-Koyanagi-Harada syndrome. Note loss of retinal pigment epithelial pigment and multiple round depigmented dots, site of previous Dalen-Fuchs nodules.

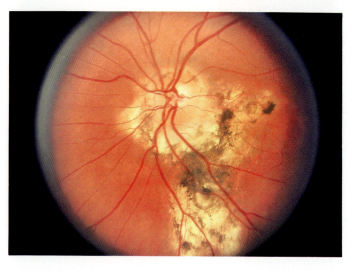

Figure 10.6. A case of geographic choroiditis.

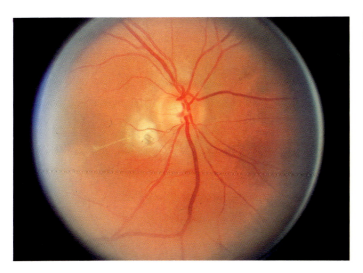

Figure 10.7. Healed nematode retinal infestation.

Laterality

Posterior uveitis may be bilateral or unilateral. In general, posterior uveitis caused by autoimmune disorders (e.g., Vogt-Koyanagi-Harada syndrome, Behcet's disease, sympathetic ophthalmia) lead to bilateral involvement with clinical manifestations in both eyes. Conditions that frequently cause unilateral disease are mostly infectious in origin and include toxoplasmosis, candidiasis, toxocariasis, acute retinal necrosis syndrome, CMV, and endogenous bacterial infection.

Onset of the Disease

The onset of posterior uveitis may be acute and sudden or chronic and insidious. Diseases of the posterior segment of the eye that may present with sudden onset include toxoplasmic retinitis, CMV retinitis, acute retinal necrosis, and bacterial infections. Most autoimmune disorders causing posterior uveitis may present with chronic and insidious onset. History of trauma is important to rule out intraocular foreign body or sympathetic ophthalmia in patients with uveitis.

Symptoms

Patients with posterior uveitis may present with decrease in vision, and this cannot be a helpful localizing symptom in patients with posterior uveitis.

Redness of the eye is seen in patients who develop diffuse uveitis in association with posterior uveitis and is seen in most patients with Behcet's, Vogt-Koyanagi-Harada syndrome, and sympathetic ophthalmia. Patients who develop posterior uveitis without involvement of the anterior segment of the eye may present with no evidence of redness of the eye (e.g., toxoplasmosis and histoplasmosis). Ocular pain is observed in patients who have acute retinal necrosis syndrome, syphilis, endogenous bacterial infection, posterior scleritis, and in rare conditions in which the optic nerve is involved. Patients with toxoplasmosis, toxocariasis, and CMV retinitis who do not have evidence of glaucoma usually present with no pain in the eye. Other non-infectious diseases that may afflict the posterior segment of the eye and are typically not associated with pain include acute multifocal placoid pigment epitheliopathy, geographic choroiditis, Vogt-Koyanagi-Harada syndrome, and Behcet's disease.

Signs of Posterior Uveitis

Signs that are important in the diagnosis of posterior uveitis include hypopyon, granulomatous uveitis, glaucoma, vitritis, morphology of the lesion, vasculitis, retinal hemorrhages, and old scars. Certain disorders of the posterior segment may present with hypopyon. This includes retinoblastoma, non-Hodgkin's lymphoma, leukemia, Behcet's disease, syphilis, toxocariasis and endogenous bacterial infections. Anterior granulomatous uveitis may be associated with conditions that affect the posterior retina and choroid, for example, patients with sarcoidosis, tuberculosis, toxoplasmosis, sporadic syphilis, endemic syphilis (Bejel), brucellosis, Vogt-Koyanagi-Harada syndrome, and sympathetic ophthalmia. All of these entities may lead to inflammatory changes in the posterior segment of the eye and are usually associated with mutton-fat keratic precipitates. Conversely, nongranulomatous anterior uveitis may be associated with Behcet's disease, acute multifocal placoid pigment epitheliopathy, reticulum cell sarcoma, and acute retinal necrosis syndrome. Secondary glaucoma may be observed in patients who have acute retinal necrosis syndrome, toxoplasmosis, tuberculosis, or sarcoidosis. Inflammation of the vitreous body may be associated with posterior uveitis. The inflammatory changes in the vitreous are caused by spillover from the inflammatory foci in the posterior segment of the eye or by active invasion by infectious agents. Inflammatory changes in the vitreous are not observed in patients with geographic choroiditis or histoplasmosis. Minimal inflammatory cells in the vitreous may be observed in patients with acute multifocal placoid pigment epitheliopathy (AMPPE), CMV, rubella, and some cases of toxoplasmosis with a small focus of infection in the retina. Conversely, severe inflammatory changes in the vitreous with marked cells and exudates may be seen in tuberculosis, brucellosis, Lyme disease, toxocariasis, syphilis, Behcet's disease, Nocardiosis, large granuloma caused by toxoplasmosis, and in patients with endogenous *Candida* or bacterial endophthalmitis.

Patients with certain diseases develop retinitis, others develop predominant choroiditis, and some diseases cause both retinitis and choroiditis. Retinitis and retinal vasculitis are seen in patients with Behcet's disease. Patients with Vogt-Koyanagi-Harada syndrome develop severe choroiditis and retinal detachment. Patients with sympathetic ophthalmia have predominant involvement of the choroid. Toxoplasmosis is a typical example causing a necrotizing retinitis with inflammation in the subjacent choroid. Furthermore, CMV, herpesvirus, rubella virus, rubeola virus, usually involve the retina primarily and cause more retinitis than choroiditis. Each of these known entities affects the retina more than it does any other structure in the posterior segment of the eye. The active lesion of toxoplasmosis is generally seen in the company of old healed pigmented retinochoroiditic scars. The vitreous is generally clouded when large lesions are observed. The lesions of cytomegalic inclusion disease affect the retina of immunologically compromised hosts. In patients with tuberculosis, the choroid is the primary target of a geographic granulomatous process that may also affect the retina. By contrast, patients with presumed ocular histoplasmosis syndrome have multiple small coinlike lesions that never cloud the overlying vitreous. Peripapillary scarring and macular lesions leading to subretinal neovascular nets may be observed. In

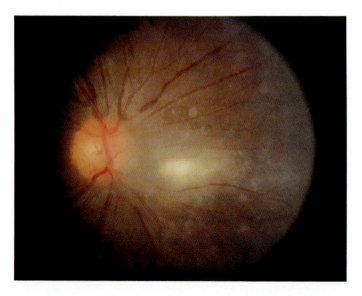

Figure 10.8. Acquired ocular toxoplasmosis in a 16-year-old female patient who developed a single focus of retinitis six weeks following systemic toxoplasmosis.

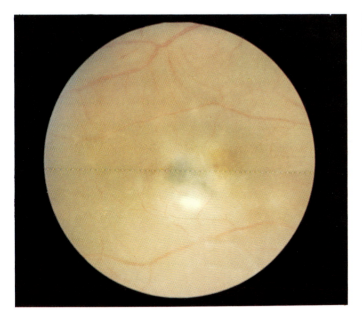

Figure 10.9. Recurrent ocular toxoplasmosis. A focus of active retinitis adjacent to a healed pigmented retino-choroiditic scar.

general there are no signs of systemic disease in patients with presumed ocular histoplasmosis syndrome; however, radiographs of the chest may show evidence of dissemination and calcific changes in the periphery of the lung fields. The active lesions in the various disorders causing posterior uveitis may vary; some are geographic, and others are punctate or nummular. Geographic lesions are seen in CMV retinitis, tuberculosis, toxocariasis, geographic choroiditis, and acute retinal necrosis syndrome. Nummular punctate or coinlike lesions are seen in patients with rubella, rubeola, Behcet's disease, AMPPE, and toxoplasma. In Vogt-Koyanagi-Harada syndrome and sympathetic ophthalmia, Dalen-Fuchs nodules are seen. Sarcoidosis affects any tissue in the eye and may show geographic lesions, retinal vasculitis, and candlewax drippings. In patients with CMV, rubella, rubeola, and acute retinal necrosis syndrome, the lesions are strictly retinal, with minimal or no inflammatory changes in the subjacent tissue. In patients with histoplasmosis, tuberculosis, syphilis, nonendemic syphilis, and cryptococcosis, the inflammatory lesions are deep choroidal and multifocal. Conversely, patients with Vogt-Koyanagi-Harada syndrome and AMPPE, the lesions are at the level of the retinal pigment epithelium. Elevated necrotic whitish lesions are seen in patients with *Candida* retinitis and toxoplasmosis. In addition, candida tend to invade the vitreous, show-

ing the string of pearls appearance in the vitreous as well as snowball-like lesions. Exudative retinal detachment is typically seen in patients with Vogt-Koyanagi-Harada and Lyme disease. Diffuse choroiditis may be seen in sympathetic ophthalmia, leukemia, tuberculosis, brucellosis, and Lyme disease.

Retinitis associated with arteritis is seen in patients with acute retinal necrosis syndrome and toxoplasmosis. A retinitis with phlebitis is seen most frequently in Behcet's disease, syphilis, CMV retinitis, and in patients with multiple sclerosis. Furthermore, patients with intermediate uveitis may show evidence of extensive retinal phlebitis in the periphery.

Cytomegalovirus infection of the retina occurs almost always in patients who are immunocompromised. Herpes simplex retinitis may be seen in association with encephalitis in the postnatal period but has been also described in healthy adults. Herpes simplex retinitis may cause necrotizing retinitis and retinal vasculitis. Herpes simplex and herpes zoster have been implicated as a cause of acute retinal necrosis syndrome. Retinal vasculitis has also been described in Lyme disease.

Posterior uveitis associated with retinal hemorrhages is seen in patients with CMV retinitis, Behcet's disease, acute retinal necrosis, and subacute sclerosing panencephalitis. Several conditions causing posterior uveitis may be associated with scars in the posterior segment of the eye. This in-

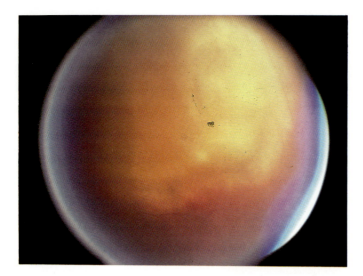

Figure 10.10. A large toxoplasmic granuloma of the posterior pole.

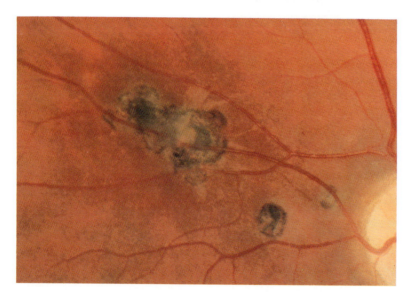

Figure 10.11. Healed toxoplasmic retinochoroiditic scars.

cludes toxocariasis, toxoplasmosis, CMV retinitis, Vogt-Koyanagi-Harada syndrome, and histoplasmosis. Each of those scars has an atypical appearance. In patients with toxocariasis, the scars consist of fibrotic or fibrovascular growth on the surface of the retina, occasionally seen pulling on the optic nerve head. In patients with toxoplasmosis the retinochoroiditic scar may represent a clump of pigment or it could be a punched-out scar surrounded by variable amounts of pigmentation. The fresh lesions of toxoplasmosis are frequently seen in the vicinity of old healed scars. Patients with CMV retinitis usually have two forms of the disease: (1) hemorrhagic form and (2) granular form. In both forms the scars of the CMV retinitis typically show no evidence of pigmentation. The healed scar appears pale and flat and sometimes geographic of various sizes. In patients with Vogt-Koyanagi-Harada syndrome, the scars are nummular, surrounded by pigment. Retinal pigment epithelial pigment migration may be seen in the aftermath of Vogt-Koyanagi-Harada syndrome with extensive loss of the pigment in the retinal pigment epithelium. The typical scars of presumed ocular histoplasmosis syndrome appear nummular with variable amounts of pigmentations around or in the scar. In patients with tuberculosis, acquired syphilis (endemic and sporadic) geographic and patchy

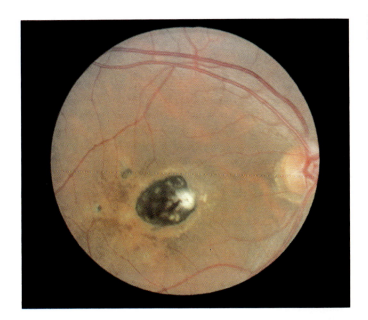

Figure 10.12. Toxoplasmic hypertrophic pigmented scar.

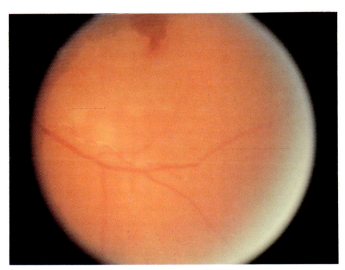

Figure 10.13. An early case of acute retinal necrosis syndrome in an immunocompetent 62-year-old man. Patient had focal retinal infiltrate, retinal arteritis, and peripheral retinal necrosis.

choroidal scars may be seen. Patients with congenital syphilis show a picture of pigmentation and depigmentation that gives a salt-and-pepper appearance to the fundus.

Behcet's disease may be associated with erythema nodosum, cutaneous phlebitis, and pustular lesions of the skin. Patients with secondary syphilis may develop maculopapular eruptions with scaling of the skin of palms and soles. Skin lesions such as erythema nodosum are observed in patients with sarcoidosis. Vitiligo and poliosis may be seen in patients with sympathetic ophthalmia and Vogt-Koyanagi-Harada syndrome. Petechial hemorrhages are ob-

served in patients with meningococcemia, who also may have meningitis caused by *Neisseria meningitidis*. Patients with AIDS may have Kaposi's sarcoma of the skin. Other viral infections such as herpes simplex, herpes zoster, Epstein–Barr (E–B) virus, rubella, and rubeola also develop typical skin lesions in the acute stages of the disease.

AIDS

Posterior uveitis may be seen in patients with AIDS. Ophthalmic manifestations in this disease are fre-

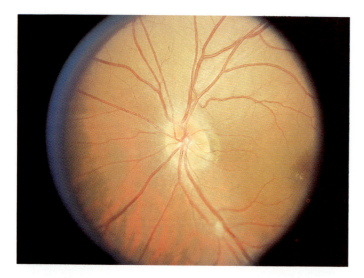

Figure 10.14. One cotton-wool spot adjacent to the inferotemporal artery in the left eye of a patient with acquired immune deficiency syndrome.

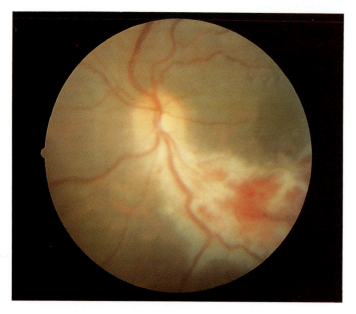

Figure 10.15. Sector juxtapapillary retinitis with retinal hemorrhages secondary to cytomegalovirus infection. Patient was a 30-year-old man who presented with a history of seeing floaters. Serum antibodies to HIV were determined and found to be positive.

quent and may have both prognostic and diagnostic significance. Clinical and histopathologic studies have certainly led to a better understanding of the ophthalmic disorders associated with this syndrome. Ocular manifestations include cotton-wool spots, retinal hemorrhages, Kaposi's sarcoma of the ocular surface and adnexa, and neuro-ophthalmic abnormalities associated with intracranial disease. In addition, patients with AIDS frequently develop infections by opportunistic organisms. Cytomegalovirus retinopathy is a blinding disease and is the most common ocular infection in patients with AIDS. Other infections that may cause ocular manifesta-

tions in patients with AIDS include *Pneumocystis carinii, Candida spp., Toxoplasma gondii, Mycobacterium avium-complex,* and *Cryptococcus.*

Diagnostic Tests for Posterior Uveitis

As mentioned earlier, the diagnostic tests for patients with posterior uveitis are used for the refinement of the entities that may manifest with similar signs and symptoms. The diagnostic tests used include A- and B-scan ultrasonography, which may help to delineate the level of retinitis and the presence of choroiditis. This is also important in assessing the thickness of the choroid in patients with sympathetic ophthalmia and the posterior sclera in posterior scleritis. Diagnostic vitrectomy may help to isolate the offensive agent or to determine the presence of specific antigens or antibodies. Serology on the vitreous specimens may be helpful to define the cause of the posterior uveitis. Viral, bacterial, and fungal cultures may be used, and the cytospin is a helpful technique for concentrating the organisms or cells for cytologic examination.

Abnormal malignant cells may be seen in masquerade syndrome and in patients with CNS lymphoma. Polymorphonuclear cells may indicate the presence of bacterial or fungal infections. The presence of eosinophils may indicate a parasitic infection in the eye such as toxocariasis. In patients with neurologic findings, a lumbar puncture may help, and the cerebrospinal fluid may be submitted for cytology and biochemical analysis. Viral and bacterial cultures are helpful. A computerized tomograph (CT) scan or magnetic resonance imaging (MRI) may be helpful to rule out CNS lymphoma or, in cases of intracranial tuberculosis or toxoplasmosis, may be helpful in ruling out intracranial tuberculoma or toxoplasmoma.

There are many other laboratory investigations to rule out systemic diseases such as syphilis, tuberculosis, and sarcoidosis. Luetic serology, purified protein derivative, and chest radiograph are performed to rule out syphilis and tuberculosis. Angiotensin-converting enzyme and lysozyme are serologic markers for sarcoidosis. Serologic tests for human immune deficiency virus, herpes simplex virus, rubella, Coxsackie virus, Epstein–Barr virus, *Borrelia,* and *Yersinia* are available and can be ordered whenever indicated. Audiometry may be helpful in assessing hearing, which may be affected in patients with Vogt-Koyanagi-Harada syndrome and sympathetic ophthalmia. Diagnostic molecular microbiology will play an important role in the diagnosis of posterior uveitis in the future.

References

1. Kraus-Mackiw E, O'Connor GR: Uveitis: Pathophysiology and therapy. New York: Thieme-Stratton, 1983.
2. Smith RE, Nozik RM: Uveitis: A clinical approach to diagnosis and management. Baltimore: Williams & Wilkins, 1983.
3. Tabbara KF: Ocular toxoplasmosis. In Duane TD (ed.): Clinical ophthalmology. Philadelphia: Harper and Row, 1987:1–23.
4. BenEzra D: Diseases of the choroid and anterior uvea. In Michaelson IC (ed.): Michaelson's textbook of the fundus of the eye, 3rd ed. Edinburgh: Churchill Livingston, 1980:435–460.
5. Aaberg TM, O'Brien WJ: Expanding ophthalmologic recognition of Epstein–Barr infections. Am J Ophthalmol 1987;104:20.
6. Tiedman JS: Epstein-Barr viral antibodies in multifocal choroiditis and panuveitis. Am J Ophthalmol 1987; 103:659.
7. Bialasiewicz AA, Ruprecht KW, Naumann GOH, Blank H: Bilateral diffuse choroiditis and exudative retinal detachments with evidence of Lyme disease. Am J Ophthalmol 1988;105:419.
8. Nussenblatt RD, Palestine AG: Uveitis fundamentals and clinical practice. Chicago: Yearbook Medical Publishers, 1989.

IV

Medical Therapy of Posterior Uveitis

Chapter 11
Therapy of Posterior Uveitis and Future Considerations

Khalid F. Tabbara

Medical Therapy of Posterior Uveitis

The success of medical treatment in patients with posterior uveitis relies on making the correct clinical diagnosis. Several important considerations must be made when therapy for posterior uveitis is contemplated. Therapeutic intervention should not be initiated before a complete history is taken, a thorough clinical evaluation is done, and laboratory testing is completed.

The following questions should be asked from the outset:

1. What is the clinical diagnosis? What is the natural course of the disease; is it short and self-limited or is it protracted and progressive? Is the disease fulminant and explosive or is it smouldering and insidious? Answers to these questions are important in determining the type of drug to be used, the dosage, and the length of therapy.
2. Is the lesion in the posterior segment of the eye reversible or irreversible? Treatment of patients with irreversible lesions such as optic atrophy has little justification. Treatment of these patients may have to be focused on symptomatology and on relieving symptoms such as pain.
3. The age of the patient should be considered in deciding the type of drug to be used, the dose, and the length of therapy.
4. Compliance and availability of the patient for clinical follow-up evaluation and surveillance are extremely important in patients with posterior uveitis. Many therapeutic measures used for the treatment of uveitis carry considerable risks. It is therefore necessary that patients who will be subjected to therapy should be reliable and available for uninterrupted clinical surveillance.
5. The objective of therapy should be well defined. In most cases it is the relief of symptoms that comes first, such as the relief of pain, photophobia, redness, and irritation. The ultimate goal is to arrest the disease process, reverse the lesions caused by the inflammatory process, and regain visual acuity.
6. The type of the drug to be used, the route, and the duration have to be decided based on the clinical observations. One has to judge the risks and benefits from such therapeutic intervention. The use of immunosuppressive agents in end-stage disease has very little justification.
7. In infectious causes of posterior uveitis, specific antimicrobial therapy should be used and immunosuppression should be avoided. Steroids should be used with caution.

In general, anterior segment inflammatory actions may be approached by topical and subconjunctival treatment with antiinflammatory agents such as corticosteroids. Posterior segment lesions have to be treated systemically with antiinfectious or antiinflammatory agents, depending on the condition and the cause of the disease. The presence of fibrin in the anterior chamber, specifically when it is seen in the angle, is an ominous sign. Such findings require vigorous topical and periocular treatment with antiinflammatory agents. In posterior segment lesions such as retinal vasculitis, delay in therapy may result in vascular occlusion and retinal necrosis. In acute conditions with severe anterior segment inflammatory reaction, one way to prevent or break the posterior synechiae that have formed during an acute attack is to give periocular injections of corticosteroids (e.g., prednisolone 1% eyedrops) every minute for 5 minutes every hour over a period of 6 hours. In addition, one should combine such therapy with a cocktail of dilating agents consisting of cocaine, homatropine, and phenylephrine. The dose of corticosteroids used topically is determined by the mode of onset of the disease, the severity of the disease, and the type of anterior segment inflammatory reaction. Intraocular fibrin, in certain conditions, may be dissolved by the use of fibrinolytic agents such as tissue plasminogen activator or streptokinase. The role of therapy is not to remove the cells and flare from the anterior chamber but, more importantly, to diminish the inflammatory reactions in the anterior segment of the eye, thus preventing further damage or destruction to the ocular structures that may lead to serious complications such as intraocular tissue adhesions, and glaucoma.

It is of crucial importance to let the patient understand, especially when the condition is chronic, that the treatment requires long-term care. The patient should also understand the risks and benefits of this therapy. Therapeutic alternatives should be presented to the patient. Informed consent should be written whenever the therapy is not approved for that particular disease or when the patient is a subject in an experimental study. Adequate time should be spent with each patient who suffers from chronic uveitis.

Corticosteroids

There are several types of corticosteroids used for combatting inflammatory reactions within the eye. Steroids are considered the mainstay for therapy of uveitis. Systemic steroids may be used in patients with autoimmune uveitis such as sympathetic ophthalmia and Vogt-Koyanagi-Harada syndrome.

Corticosteroid therapy may be given orally or intravenously. Patients with sympathetic ophthalmia or Vogt-Koyanagi-Harada syndrome may develop severe peripapillary choroiditis leading to hyperemia of the optic nerve head. This, if not appropriately treated, may lead to damage of the optic nerve head. Early diagnosis and prompt treatment of such conditions may prevent some of the complications that lead to loss of vision. In certain severe forms of Vogt-Koyanagi-Harada disease with exudative retinal detachment, one may give the patient pulse therapy of methylprednisolone intravenously over a few days. This can be followed by the administration of oral corticosteroids such as prednisone. It is believed that high-dose prednisone therapy is an effective approach for the treatment of severe noninfectious posterior uveitis. Prednisone therapy may be started at a dosage level of 1 to 1.5 mg/kg daily. The treatment has to be combined with antacids and calcium supplements, particularly for those who are placed on long-term therapy. When the disease is under control, the systemic oral prednisolone therapy can be tapered, and when the patient's condition is under control and in remission, he or she may be placed on alternate-day prednisone therapy consisting of 20 to 40 mg orally every other day. In certain patients, the use of systemic corticosteroid therapy may have to be combined with cytotoxic agents or cyclosporine.

Cytotoxic Agents

Only a few cytotoxic agents are used in the treatment of inflammatory conditions of the eye, including noninfectious chronic posterior uveitis. It may take several days or sometimes weeks for patients with noninfectious posterior uveitis to be clinically treated. This lag period may result in irreversible damage to certain ocular structures and may defeat the principles of early therapeutic intervention. Patients with evidence of acute retinal vasculitis may benefit from immunosuppressive therapy. Certain cytotoxic agents may take 1 to 2 weeks before they appear to be clinically active. In certain instances, we have found that the use of cyclosporine, which is effective in the early treatment of certain forms of vasculitis, may be more suitable than the use of cytotoxic agents in patients with noninfectious disorders of the posterior uveitis. The commonly used cytotoxic agents in noninfectious causes and immunologically mediated causes of uveitis include:

A. Alkylating agents
1. Cyclophosphamide
2. Chlorambucil
B. Antimetabolites
1. Azathioprine
2. Methotrexate
3. Fluorouracil

The New Horizon of Immunologic Intervention

The current therapeutic regimen available for the treatment of autoimmune disorders affecting the posterior segment of the eye were developed before our clear knowledge of the mechanisms involved in immunologic activation and interactions.

Recent developments in the fields of ophthalmology and molecular biology have greatly influenced our understanding of the relationship between self and non-self. The diversity of the immune system and the intricate network of immunologic reactions are starting to become recognized, from the cytokines to the lymphokines, and from cell receptors to immune factors. Workers in the field of autoimmunity are becoming more and more intrigued by the microcosms of the vast immunologic network. Since the dawn of medical history, in 1900, Ehrlich described the so-called "horror autoxicus" phenomenon, suggesting that the immune system does not normally react to self-antigens. Burnett, however, suggested that the lymphocytes that react with self-antigens are eliminated early in the development of the immune system. Unfortunately, modern immunology and recent advances in the field have challenged these two hypotheses, and both great immunologists were proven to be incorrect. Researchers in the field of immunology have recently recognized the phenomenon of self-recognition and the cell surface antigen of host cells, referred to as major histocompatibility (MHC) molecules. This recognition of cells was once considered to be harmful and a sign of autoaggression leading to tissue injury and disease. The concept, however, was later modified by observations showing that autoreactive T and B cells are present in normal individuals without evidence of disease. A distinction between autorecognition, autoreactivity, and autoimmune disease began to emerge. The word *autoimmune* is linked inextricably to disease. It is now believed that recognition of MHC self molecules by T cells during and after development is the driving force shaping and building the T cell repertoire and taskforce. The lines between physiologic and pathologic autoreactivity and autoimmunity are subtle. Autoimmunity may have a physiologic role or may be a product of unrelated phenomena of immunologic challenge. The interaction between immunologically competent lymphocytes involved in the recognition and killing of virus-infected cells may be dependent on the mutual recognition of cell surface markers and may represent a form of selective localized autoimmunity. Similarly, the response to antiidiotypic antibodies appear as a natural, normal, physiologic form of autoreactivity and autoimmunity.

Idiotypes are unique antigenic regions of immunoglobulins that correspond to antibody-combining sites. They are also present on lymphocyte cell surface. Self-reactive autoantibodies such as rheumatoid factor may be produced by vaccination or by challenge with polysaccharides of certain bacteria. Antigen-specific suppressor T cells are called on to suppress the production of the autoantibodies. It is therefore conceded that the cells of the immune system are charged with the task of discriminating between self and nonself under threat of immunologic self-reactivity and impending self-destruction.

There are several important factors that lead to the immunopathogenesis of autoimmune disease. These factors include genetic predisposition, environmental factors, hormonal factors, nonspecific polyclonal activation by antigens or similar substances, idiotypic antibodies, and molecular mimicry. In brief, autoimmune disorders represent a state of immunologic disregulation. The extraordinary intertwining of events in the intricate immunologic network is far from being straightforward. It is still conceptually valid, however, to simplify these potential mechanisms in the immunopathogenesis of autoimmune disease. The pillars for future therapy of autoimmune disorders rest on immunologic intervention. Future specific therapeutic intervention modalities will soon be in the hands of ophthalmologists. We are now moving from the age of nonspecific immunologic suppression and cytotoxic therapy to an age of selective inhibition of certain undesired immunopathologic pathways. Several future therapeutic modalities in immunologic intervention will have to be developed based on our current understanding of the immunologic network.

Nonspecific Immunologic Intervention

The current therapeutic modalities, consisting of corticosteroids as well as other immunosuppressive and antiinflammatory agents, share the fundamental disadvantage of not being able to distinguish between physiologic and pathologic immune response. Thus, these therapeutic modalities should be used as a last resort during the exacerbation of the disease, whereas the pathologic response must be blocked to prevent irreversible damage to the tissues. Recently, immune nonspecific modalities for immunologic intervention have been developed. The use of monoclonal antibodies directed to monomorphic components of CD3 of the T-cell receptor complex is one example. These monoclonal antibodies are currently used in the prevention and treatment of acute renal allograph rejection. This treatment is effective for a limited period. The CD3 antibodies, however, can induce severe side effects and are not good for use in autoimmune diseases. The somewhat more selective approach is to address the interleukin-2 receptors of the T lymphocytes. One can use either anti–interleukin-2 receptor antibodies or interleukin-2 toxin conjugates. This may appear to be more selective than the monoclonal antibodies targeted against CD3, because it allows the removal of activated lymphocytes, sparing only the nonactivated lymphocytes. Cyclosporine, however, has a selective effect on the T-cell activation by inhibiting the cytokine gene transcription of interleukin-2. Another future possibility is the use of monoclonal antibodies directed against CD4 and CD8 molecules expressed by the lymphocytes (binds to MHC II) as well as the lymphocyte function–associated molecules (LFA1) and CD2, which bind to MHC I.

Blocking of the Binding Site of the Major Histocompatibility Complex

It is presumed that disease-associated HLA Class II molecules have the capacity to bind autoantigens and present them to the T cells. This mechanism, under appropriate environmental conditions, may perpetuate the autoimmune process and maintain the disease. One future possible therapeutic approach to prevent activation of Class II restricted autoreactive T lymphocytes is the administration of the anti-MHC Class II antibodies. One drawback of this approach is the immunogenicity of the antibody molecules, preventing long-term therapy. An alternative therapeutic approach could include the blocking of the MHC-binding site by certain compatible peptides. The inhibition of T-cell activation by blocking the binding site of antigenic peptides to Class II molecules may prevent the induction of autoimmune diseases, as in experimental autoimmune encephalitis of mice. This therapeutic approach may lead to the development of a new generation of immunosuppressive and immunomodulating agents.

Idiotypes

Antiidiotypic treatment can be provided in the future for the treatment of autoimmune disorders. Antiidiotypic antibodies directed against T-cell receptors and B-cell receptors may be considered reasonable therapeutic modalities. In certain experimental animals, antiidiotypic antibodies recognizing the T cells mediating the experimental autoimmune encephalitis in mice have been demonstrated to prevent the disease induced by the injection of myelin basic protein. Anti–cell receptor idiotypes may downregulate the T-cell receptors or, if antibodies are conjugated to toxins, they may delete and eliminate the autoreactive T-cell clones.

Induction of Autoantigenic-Specific Tolerance

Antigen-specific tolerance or suppression is a phenomenon that has no molecular explanation so far. TGF-β (Transformation growth factor-beta) may play a role in the induction of tolerance following oral feeding. Future experimental studies may elucidate the mechanisms involved in this phenomenon. It is conceptually appealing that induction of tolerance will be a future therapeutic approach and strategy for autoimmune disease causing uveitis. Oral feeding of specific antigens appears to induce tolerance in certain animal models of autoimmune diseases.

• • • • • •

Summary

Considering our current understanding of immunologic network, the main objectives of our therapeutic modalities will be to attempt to educate and train the deranged immune system to avoid reactivity with self by giving it instructions to distinguish self from nonself. This approach remains impractical, but other options are available, including the induction of tolerance or specific suppression to the autoantigen, deletion or elimination of autoreactive cell, blocking of the disease-associated HLA Class II molecules, and the nonselective immunologic intervention by the inhibition of interleukin-2 with the use of cyclosporine or specific monoclonal antibodies directed against the interleukin-2 receptors. It has been recognized that future therapeutic modalities will have to take into consideration the clinical situation and underlying cause and pathogenesis of the disease process. Successive generations of immunologic agents will have to be aimed at high efficacy, selectivity, and safety. Current therapeutic strategies are aimed at suppression of the inflammatory reactions in a nonselective manner. It is becoming possible to match a given autoimmune disease with an appropriate treatment, depending on the pathogenesis of the disease and the immunologic mechanisms involved.

Chapter 12
Cyclosporine in Posterior Uveitis

Khalid F. Tabbara

Cyclosporine (CsA, Sandimmun®) is a cyclic undecapeptide (11 amino acids) having a molecular weight of 1202. There is an amino acid at C9 that has not been previously identified and appears to be essential for the biologic activity of the compound. Cyclosporine contains alpha-aminobutyric acid residue at position 2, whereas four other related polypeptides have different amino acids at this position. Cyclosporin C has threonine at position 2, and Cyclosporin B has alanine, Cyclosporin D has valine, and Cyclosporin G has L-nor-valine. Seven of the 11 amino acids are N-methylated, making the compound hydrophobic. Cyclosporine has been shown to be an effective agent in prolonging the survival of allogenic transplant in humans and in experimental animals. Cyclosporine inhibits the development of cell-mediated reactions, including delayed cutaneous hypersensitivity, allograft immunity, graft-versus-host disease, experimental allergic encephalomyelitis, retinal-S–induced uveitis, Freund's adjuvant arthritis, and T-cell–dependent antibody production.

Mechanism of Action of Cyclosporine

Cyclosporine acts in the basic events that lead to lymphocytic activation. CsA interferes with the synthesis and the release of interleukin-2 (IL-2). CsA does not inhibit T-cell antigen recognition and has no effect on transmembrane signaling. It also does not inhibit antigen-induced activation of protein kinase C and the subsequent increase in intracellular calcium. CsA can diffuse passively through the cell membrane and binds to the cytoplasmic cytosolic protein, cyclophillin. CsA has been shown to inhibit certain chemotactic factors for leukocytes and, specifically, eosinophils. CsA then can inhibit transcription of messenger RNA involved in the synthesis of a variety of lymphokines with high-affinity binding to the transcription factors of IL-2 promoter at concentrations similar to those found in vitro. CsA also inhibits the synthesis of IL-2 at high concentrations. Expression of major histocompatibility complex (MHC) gene products are significantly reduced by CsA. It acts reversibly and specifically on lymphocytes and, unlike cytotoxic agents, it does not depress hematopoiesis and does not inhibit phagocytic cell functions. Patients on CsA have less incidence of infections than patients receiving other immunosuppressive treatment. CsA has also been shown to inhibit chemotaxis of polymorphonuclear, especially eosinophils

Ocular Pharmacokinetics

After an oral dose of CsA, peak blood concentrations are achieved within 6 hours. The absolute bioavailability of the oral forms (capsules or suspension) is 20% to 50% at the steady state. The main distribution of CsA is extravascular. It is estimated that within the blood 41% to 58% is found in the erythrocytes and 33% to 47% is present in plasma. CsA is metabolized into more than 15 metabolites and is eliminated primarily in the bile, whereas 6% of the oral dose is excreted in the urine.

Cyclosporine has been used in the treatment of various disorders leading to endogenous uveitis.[1-38] The drug displays a wide range of interpatient pharmacokinetic variability, and its use may be associated with nephrotoxicity and hepatotoxicity. The therapeutic window is narrow, and over the past decade the dosage to maintain a therapeutic level with safety has been defined with relative precision. The risk/benefit ratio in patients receiving CsA, however, should be weighed carefully, and the therapy must be monitored closely.

Cyclosporine penetration into the aqueous of patients with uveitis was studied by Palestine and associates[28] and was found to range between 13 and 125 ng/mL, with a mean of 44 ng/mL. We studied the trough aqueous level of CsA among five patients with Behcet's disease receiving 5 mg/kg/day.[33] We found a mean trough level of 41 ng/mL with a range of 26 to 67 ng/mL after an oral dosage of 5 mg/kg/day. The ocular bioavailability of CsA was studied in experimental animals.[34] We assessed the ocular tissue absorption of CsA after oral administration among albino and pigmented rabbits.[39] The CsA mean blood level was 574 ng/mL in pigmented and 448 ng/mL in albino rabbits. There again was no detectable CsA level in the aqueous and vitreous, and there was no statistically significant difference between the CsA levels in the corneas of the pigmented and albino rabbits. The iris tissue CsA level was significantly higher in pigmented rabbits when compared with the albino rabbits ($P < 0.01$).[39] The CsA level in the retina/choroid was significantly higher in the pigmented rabbits when compared with the albino rabbits, however. This study has shown CsA to concentrate in the pigmented layers of the uvea. In patients with uveitis, the concentration of CsA in the uveal tissue is highly desirable. The bioavailability of CsA in the uvea, the target tissue of therapy in uveitis, has great clinical significance.

Cyclosporine in Uveitis

There are four major groups of ocular disorders in which CsA has been used, these include (1) corneal transplantation, (2) ocular surface disorders, (3) intraocular inflammation, and (4) ocular disorders associated with skin diseases. The most important

Table 12.1. Uveitis Disorders Treated with Cyclosporine

Behcet's disease
Sympathetic ophthalmia
Vogt-Koyanagi-Harada syndrome
Birdshot retinochoroidopathy
Serpiginous choroiditis
Intermediate uveitis
Sarcoidosis
Retinal vasculitis
Other endogenous noninfectious uveitis

group of patients are those suffering from endogenous noninfectious uveitis. This includes patients with autoimmune disorders. Table 12.1 demonstrates the ocular disorders in which cyclosporine has been found to be an effective therapeutic modality. CsA has been used in the treatment of endogenous uveitis at variable therapeutic levels.

Behcet's disease is a chronic systemic inflammatory disorder of unknown cause. It is characterized by recurrent oral or genital ulcer, neurologic and ocular manifestations, skin lesions, and arthritis. The objective of therapy in these patients is to prevent the structural damage that may occur during the episodes of inflammation. Our group has treated 24 patients with Behcet's disease. All patients had definite Behcet's characterized by the presence of uveitis, aphthous ulcers, genital ulcers, and skin lesions. All patients had evidence of retinal vasculitis with or without optic nerve involvement. The ocular changes in our patients included a nongranulomatous anterior uveitis with vitreous exudates, retinal infiltrates, retinal vasculitis, and occlusive vascular disease of the retina. Historical cases of Behcet's with retinal vasculitis and papillitis who were treated with other therapeutic modalities (steroids and chlorambucil) became blind within 5 years after the onset of the disorder. We have followed these patients for a mean period of 5 years. Our patients with retinal vasculitis received low-dose CsA consisting of 5 mg/kg/day or less for a mean period of 4 weeks. The dosage of CsA was tapered when the patient responded to treatment and the inflammatory reaction was under control. The treatment was given intermittently during recurrences of the disease.

In open clinical trials, Nussenblatt and associates[21] treated patients with bilateral sight-threatening posterior uveitis of noninfectious origin who had not responded to steroids or cytotoxic agent therapy. Eight patients were treated with cyclosporine and all patients were started at a dosage level of 10 mg/kg/day. Seven of the eight patients showed evidence of improvement in visual acuity and disappearance of ocular inflammatory disease. These seven patients included two patients with Behcet's disease who also had improvement in their nonocular symptoms. In every patient there was evidence of an increase in blood creatinine and urea nitrogen. Palestine and associates treated nine patients younger than 16 years of age with chronic intermediate or posterior uveitis with CsA patients who had shown previous resistance to high doses of systemic corticosteroids.[26] Oral therapy was given at a dosage level of 8 mg/kg/day, and the dose was adjusted based on the clinical response and toxicity. Therapy was continued for a period of 3 to 12 months. Improvement in vision and decrease in the intraocular inflammatory reaction was noted in eight of the nine patients. Nephrotoxicity was uncommon in their group of patients, and only two patients manifested elevated serum creatinine. Hirsutism was the main problem and was observed in five patients. Mild anemia was noted in five patients, gingivitis in three, and paresthesia in three. In addition, two patients had gastrointestinal disturbances. This study suggests that children with posterior uveitis may be considered as candidates for treatment with systemic CsA. This is also important because of the growth retardation that may occur with the long-term use of corticosteroid.

In an open clinical trial, Akazawa and co-workers[1] treated nine patients with severe ocular manifestations of Behcet's disease resistant to conventional therapy.[1] They started their patients on 10 mg/kg/day. The duration of therapy ranged from 2 to 5 months. Visual acuity in their group of patients improved, as well as the oral aphthous lesions and the erythema nodosum. In another open clinical trial in the United Kingdom, Graham and associates treated nine patients with severe refractory posterior uveitis.[13] Four patients had Behcet's disease, one had HLA B27–related arthritis and uveitis, three had idiopathic retinal vasculitis, and one had sarcoidosis. CsA had beneficial ocular effects in all patients in early stages of treatment with an improvement in the visual acuity and decrease in the severity of inflammatory reactions. The relapse rate and the need for additional steroid treatment were reduced in all patients. Similar open clinical trials were conducted in other countries, including Turkey (Muftuoglu), Israel (BenEzra), Australia (Wakefield), Egypt (Elmarkabi), United Kingdom (Towler, Binder), and Spain (Diaz-Llopiz).[4,5,10,11,19,37,38] Two double-masked clinical trials comparing CsA with colchicine (Masuda)[18] and CsA with conventional therapy (BenEzra)[4] were carried out on patients with intraocular inflammation who were suffering from Behcet's disease. In the study by BenEzra, et al.,[4] patients were randomized into two groups: one group received Sandimmun 10 mg/kg/day, which was slowly tapered to 5 mg/kg/day as soon as the intraocular inflammation was controlled. The other group of patients were treated with steroids or chlorambucil (17 with steroids and 3 with chlorambucil). Two years after treatment was started, eighteen of the twenty patients showed stable or improved ocular condition. In the group receiving conventional therapy, eight patients had to be removed from the masked evaluation because of worsening of their ocular condition; they were placed on CsA. There was marked and significant improvement in their ocular condition. In Japan, Masuda and his associates[18] studied, in a double-masked clinical trial, the effects of CsA in Behcet's disease. These effects were assessed in a randomized double-blind study including forty-seven patients in the CsA group and forty-nine patients in the colchicine group. Thirty-six patients were entered in a long-term open trial. CsA was initiated at a dosage of 10 mg/kg/day, and the dose was adjusted according to the clinical symptoms and adverse effects. This study showed that CsA was more effective than colchicine in the treatment of uveitis, oral ulcers, skin lesions, and genital ulceration. Efficacy did not change during the long-term treatment.

Cyclosporine also was found to be effective in the treatment of serpiginous choroiditis, and in birdshot retinochoroidopathy. In patients with Behcet's disease, CsA can be used as the first line of treatment, especially if there is evidence of threatening vasculitis. Adult patients with posterior uveitis of noninfectious origin may be started on CsA 4 to 5 mg/kg/day orally (Table 12.2). Children can tolerate higher dosage, 5 to 7 mg/kg/day. Patients should be monitored for renal functions, including deter-

Table 12.2. Cyclosporine* in Uveitis

Initial Dose:
Children: Cyclosporine (oral) 5–7 mg/kg/day
Adults: Cyclosporine (oral) 3–5 mg/kg/day with or without
  prednisolone (oral) 0.5 mg/kg/day
Maintenance dosage 1–3 mg/kg/day. Dosage to be tapered
  by 0.5 mg/kg every week with improvement of
  clinical findings or in cases of major adverse effects
  (e.g., nephrotoxicity).

*Sandimmun Capsules, 25-mg/capsules. Sandimmun suspension contains 100 mg/mL cyclosporine.

mination of blood urea nitrogen and creatinine, initially once per week. If the dosage has to be increased, it should *not* be increased more than 7.5 mg/kg/day, and renal functions should be closely monitored weekly. The dosage of CsA may be kept at 5 mg/kg/day for a period of 3 to 4 weeks, which later can be tapered down based on the clinical response and adverse effects. Table 12.3 gives the adverse effects of oral CsA. CsA can be given at a low dose (<3 mg/kg/day) for prolonged periods. We have maintained patients with uveitis on low-dose CsA for a period of 2 to 3 years without any clinical evidence of nephrotoxicity. Remember that there are several drugs that may interact with CsA. Certain drugs may increase or decrease the level of cyclosporine by competitive inhibition or by induction of hepatic enzymes (Cytochrome P450). Table 12.4 shows the drugs that may interact with cyclosporine. The dosage of cyclosporine should be adjusted if other drugs are used simultaneously.

Table 12.3. Adverse Effects of Systemic Cyclosporine

A. Paresthesia
  Gastrointestinal discomfort
  Malaise
  Fatigue
  Headache
  Dysmenorrhea
  Muscle cramps
  Generalized weakness
B. Hypertrichosis
  Nephrotoxicity
  Hypertension
  Gingival hyperplasia
  Hepatotoxicity
  Anemia
  Tremor

Table 12.4. Drug Interactions with Cyclosporine

Drugs increasing blood level of cyclosporine
  Calcium channel–blocking agents (Nicardipine,
    Diltiazem, Verapamil)
  Ketoconazole
  Erythromycin
  Doxycycline
  Oral contraceptives
Drugs that may decrease the blood level of cyclosporine
  Barbiturates
  Carbamazepine
  Phenytoin
  Metamizole
  Rifampicin
  Nafcillin
Drugs that potentiate nephrotoxicity
  Diclofenac
  Aminoglycosides
  Amphotericin B
  Trimethoprim
Drugs that augment gingival hyperplasia
  Nifedipine
  Epanutin
Other: CsA reduces clearance of prednisone

References

1. Whitcup SM, Salvo EC, Nussenblatt RB: Combined cyclosporine and corticosteroid therapy for sight saving. Uveitis in Behcet's disease. Am J Ophthalmol 1994; 118:39–45.
2. Arocker-Mettinger E, Grabner G: Zur Problematik der intermediaren Uveitis (Intermediate uveitis: clinical findings and treatment.) Klin Mbl Augenheik 1989;194: 249–251.
3. BenEzra D, Maftzir G, de Courten C, Timonen P: Ocular penetration of Cyclosporin A. III: The human eye. Br J Ophthalmol 1990;74:350–352.
4. BenEzra D, Cohen, E: Treatment and visual prognosis in Behcet's disease. Br J Ophthalmol 1986;70:589.
5. Binder AI, Graham EM, Sanders MD, et al.: Cyclosporine A in the treatment of severe Behcet's uveitis Br J Rheumatol 1987;26:285–291.
6. Deray G, Baumelou B, Le Hoang P, et al.: Enhancement of cyclosporine nephrotoxicity by diuretic therapy. Clin Nephrol 1989;32:47.
7. Deray G, Le Hoang P, Aupetit B, et al.: Enhancement of cyclosporine A nephrotoxicity by diclofenac. Clin Nephrol 1987;27:213–214.
8. Chavis PS, Antonios S, Tabbara KF: Cyclosporine effects on optic nerve and retinal vasculitis in Behcet's disease. Documenta Ophthalmologica 1992;80:133–142.
9. De Vries J, Baarsma GS, Zaal MJW, et al.: Cyclosporine in the treatment of severe chronic idiopathic uveitis. Br J Ophthalmol 1990;74:344–349.

10. Diaz-Llopis M, Cervera M, Menezo JL: Cyclosporine A treatment of Behcet's disease: A long-term study. Curr Eye Res 1990;9(Suppl.):17–23.

11. El-Markabi H, Malaty A, Assad-Khalil S: Treatment of non-infectious endogenous uveitis with cyclosporine A. Bull Ophthalmol Soc Egypt 1989;82:327–333.

12. French-Constant C, Wolman R, James DG: Cyclosporine in Behcet's disease (Letter to the Editor). Lancet 1983;II:454.

13. Graham EM, Sanders MD, James DG, et al.: Cyclosporine A in the treatment of posterior uveitis. Trans Ophthalmol Soc UK 1985;104:146–151.

14. Harada T, Murakami K, Niwa M, Awaya S: Combination treatment with cyclosporine and bromocriptine in Behcet's disease, in Usui M, Ohno S, Aoki K (eds): Ocular immunology today. Proceedings of the 5th International Symposium on the Immunology and Immunopathology of the Eye, Tokyo, Japan, March 13–15, 1990. Amsterdam: Excerpta Medica, 1990:479–482.

15. Harada T, Sugita K, Saito A, Awaya S: Traitement des uveites severes par la ciclosporine. A Ophthalmologica (Basel) 1987;195:21–25.

16. Jobin D, Thillaye B, de Kozak Y, et al.: Severe retinochoroidopathy: Variations of humoral and cellular immunity to S-antigen in a longitudinal study. Curr Eye Res 1990;9(Suppl.):91–96.

17. Karjalainen K: Cyclosporin A treatment for chronic uveitis associated with retinitis. Acta Ophthalmol (Kbh) 1984;62:631–635.

18. Masuda K, Nakajima A, Urayama A, et al.: Double-masked trial of cyclosporin versus colchicine and long-term open study of cyclosporin in Behcet's disease. Lancet 1989;I:1093–1096.

19. Muftuoglu AU, Pazarli H, Yurdakul S, et al.: Short term cyclosporine A treatment of Behcet's disease. Br J Ophthalmol 1987;71:387–390.

20. Nussenblatt RB, Palestine AG, Rook AH, et al.: Treatment of intraocular inflammatory disease with cyclosporin A. Lancet 1983;II:235–238.

21. Nussenblatt RB, Palestine AG, Chan CC: Cyclosporin A therapy in the treatment of intraocular inflammatory disease resistant to systemic corticosteroids and cytotoxic agents. Am J Ophthalmol 1983;96:275–282.

22. Nussenblatt RB: Cyclosporin therapy for endogenous uveitis (Abstract 79). Acta Ophthalmol (Kbh) 1984;163(Suppl.):106–107.

23. Nussenblatt RB, Palestine AG, Chan CC: Cyclosporin therapy for uveitis: Long-term follow up. J Ocular Pharmacol 1985;1:369–382.

24. Nussenblatt RB, Palestine AG, Chan CC, et al.: Effectiveness of cyclosporine therapy for Behcet's disease. Arthritis Rheum 1985;28:671–679.

25. Palestine AG, Austin HA, Balow JE, et al.: Nephrotoxicity of cyclosporine (Correspondence). N Engl J Med 1986;315:1292.

26. Palestine AG, Nussenblatt RB, Chan CC: Cyclosporine therapy of uveitis in children (1st International Congress on Uveitis) (Abstract 80). Acta Ophthalmol (Kbh) 1984;(Suppl. 163):107.

27. Palestine AG, Nussenblatt RB, Chan CC: Side effects of systemic cyclosporine in patients not undergoing transplantation. Am J Med 1984;77:652–656.

28. Palestine AG, Nussenblatt RB, Chan CC: Cyclosporine penetration into the anterior chamber and cerebrospinal fluid. Am J Ophthalmol 1985;99:210–211.

29. Palestine AG, Roberge F, Charous BL, et al.: The effect of cyclosporine on immunization with tetanus and keyhole limpet hemocyanin (KLH) in humans. J Clin Immunol 1985;5:115–121.

30. Sanders MD, James DG, Graham E, et al.: Cyclosporine in Behcet's disease (Letter to the Editor). Lancet 1983;II:454–455.

31. Secchi AG, Tognon MS, Maselli C: Cyclosporine A in the treatment of serpiginous choroiditis. Int Ophthalmol 1990;14:395–399.

32. Svenson K, Bohman SO, Hallgren R: Renal interstitial fibrosis and vascular changes: Occurrence in patients with autoimmune disease treated with cyclosporine. Arch Intern Med 1986;146:2007–2010.

33. Tabbara KF, Gee S, Alvarez H, Cooper H: Intraocular penetration of cyclosporine, in Ferraz de Oliveira LN (ed): Ophthalmology Today. Elsevier Science Publishers, 1988:383–384.

34. Tabbara KF, Gee S, Alvarez H: Ocular bioavailability of cyclosporine. Transplant Proc 1988;XX(2 Suppl 2):656–659.

35. Towler HMA, Whiting PH, Forrester JV: Combination low dose cyclosporin A and steroid therapy in chronic intraocular inflammation. Eye 1990;4:514–520.

36. Towler HMA, Cliffe AM, Whiting PH, Forrester JF: Low dose cyclosporine A therapy in chronic posterior uveitis. Eye (Lond.) 1989;3:282–287.

37. Wakefield D, McCluskey P: Cyclosporine therapy for severe scleritis. Br J Ophthalmol 1989;73:743–746.

38. Wakefield D, McCluskey P, Reece G: Cyclosporine therapy in Vogt-Koyanagi-Harada disease. Aust N Z J Ophthalmol 1990;18(2):137–142.

39. Tabbara KF, El-Sayed YM, Cooper H, Nowailaty S: Ocular bioavailability of cyclosporin in pigmented and albino rabbits. In Recent Advances in Uveitis Proceedings of the Third International Symposium on Uveitis. Dernouchamps JP, Verougstraete C, Caspers-Velu L, Tassignon MJ (eds). Kugler Publications, 1993:501–507.

V
Summary and Conclusions

Chapter 13
Diagnosis and Laboratory Workup of Posterior Uveitis: Summary

Khalid F. Tabbara

The differential diagnosis of posterior uveitis includes the following entities.

I. **Viral infections:** AIDS, CMV, Herpes simplex, Herpes zoster, SSPE
II. **Bacterial infections:** Tuberculosis, Treponema, *Nocardia*
III. **Parasitic infections:** *Toxoplasma, Toxocara, Onchocerca*
IV. **Fungal infections:** *Candida, Histoplasma, Cryptococcus*
V. **Autoimmune diseases:** Vogt-Koyanagi-Harada syndrome, Behcet's disease, birdshot retinochoroidopathy
VI. **Diseases of unknown cause:** Sarcoidosis, Geographic choroidopathy, AMPPE

The diagnosis of posterior uveitis can be established in most cases on the basis of: (1) the morphology of the lesion; (2) the mode of onset and course of the disease; and (3) the association with other systemic diseases. Laboratory tests are mainly of use in the refinement of diagnosis or in the elimination of certain diagnoses that might otherwise need to be considered. (Table 13.1).

I. VIRAL INFECTIONS

A. **Clinical Findings:** Cotton-wool spots, microaneurysms, retinal hemorrhages
   Laboratory Tests: HIV antibodies
B. **CMV Retinitis**
   1. **Clinical Findings:** Fine fibrinoid debris on the corneal endothelium, mild vitritis, yellow-white slowly progressive retinitis occurring in any areas of the retina; there are two major forms: (a) hemorrhagic form, and (b) granular form. Other findings include papillitis, periphlebitis, and rhegmatogenous retinal detachment. The disease is progressive without treatment.
   2. **Laboratory Tests:** CMV antibody test is not helpful. Virus cultures may be obtained from the blood, urine, or from the vitreous on fibroblast cell lines. The diagnosis of CMV retinitis is made on clinical grounds.
C. **Herpes Simplex and Varicella–Zoster Retinitis (Acute Retinal Necrosis Syndrome)**
   1. **Clinical Findings:** Moderate to marked vitritis, yellow-white peripheral necrotizing retinitis sparing the posterior pole, edema of the optic nerve head with retinal arthritis, retinal hemorrhage. The disease is bilateral in two-thirds of the cases, and the retinitis undergoes resolution within 5 weeks. Rhegmatogenous retinal detachment is common.
   2. **Laboratory Tests:** Patients have detectable antibody titers for either herpes simplex virus or herpes zoster virus. Herpes virus may be cultured

Table 13.1. Diagnostic Tests for Patients with Posterior Uveitis

Disease	Diagnostic Workup
I. INFECTIONS	
A. Viral Infections	Antiviral (HSV, VZV, CMV) antibodies, HIV antibodies, chorioretinal biopsy specimen for histopathologic evaluation and viral isolation, PCR*.
B. Bacterial Infections	
1. Tuberculosis	Chest radiograph, purified protein derivative, skin test, isolation of *Mycobacterium tuberculosis* from vitreous or chorioretinal biopsy specimens, PCR.
2. Syphilis	FTA-ABS, VDRL, treponemal hemagglutination test (TPHA)
3. Nocardiosis	Chest radiograph, blood culture, isolation of bacteria from ocular specimens, lumbar puncture with analysis of cerebrospinal fluid (CSF) (If central nervous system [CNS] is involved)
4. Brucellosis	IgG and IgM antibodies to *Brucella spp.,* isolation of the organism from ocular specimens or other sites
5. Lyme borreliosis	IgG and IgM antibodies to *Borrelia burgdorferi* (ELISA, indirect fluorescent antibody [IFA] test)
C. Parasitic Infections	
1. Toxoplasmosis	IgG and IgM antibodies to *Toxoplasma gondii,* isolation of the organisms from lymph nodes of patients with acquired toxoplasmosis or from ocular specimens, PCR.
2. Toxocariasis	Antibodies to *Toxocara spp.*
3. Onchocerciasis	Skin-snip biopsy to determine number of microfilariae
D. Fungal Infections	
1. Candidiasis	Isolation of *Candida spp.* from ocular specimens
2. Cryptococcosis	Isolation of the organism by culture fluids or cerebrospinal fluid, dark-field examination after India ink stain. Detection of Cryptococcal antigens in CSF or ocular fluids
3. Histoplasmosis	Histoplasmin skin test
4. Aspergillosis	Isolation of the organisms from ocular specimens
II. AUTOIMMUNE DISEASES	
A. Behcet's disease	HLA typing for HLA-B51, skin test
B. Retinal vasculitis	Complete blood count (CBC), erythrocyte sedimentation rate (ESR), VRDL, FTA-ABS, TPHA, total serum protein, Protein electrophoresis, C3, C4, angiotensin, converting enzyme, lysozyme, antinuclear antibodies, PPD skin test, chest radiograph, anticardiolipin antibodies
C. Birdshot retinochoroid-opathy	HLA-A29
D. Vogt-Koyanagi-Harada syndrome	Audiogram, EEG, lumbar puncture, CSF cytology, protein determination, HLA DR4 HLA DQA1* 0301 (class II Antigen) and DR53
E. Sympathetic ophthalmia	Audiogram, computerized tomography (CT) scan if indicated, HLA class II Antigen DQA1. 0301
III. TUMORS	
A. Reticulum cell sarcoma (histiocytic lymphoma)	CT scan, magnetic resonance imaging (MRI), tissue biopsy specimen to confirm the diagnosis by histopathology
B. Leukemia	CBC, bone marrow biopsy, hematologic workup
C. Metastatic lesions	Chest radiograph, skeletal series, workup as indicated
IV. DISEASES OF UNKNOWN CAUSES	
A. Sarcoidosis	Chest radiograph, serum lysozyme, angiotensin-converting enzyme, lacrimal gland biopsy (specimen subjected to histopathologic evaluation) conjunctival nodule biopsy, skin test to confirm anergy, calcium, phosphorous, protein and albumin/globulin ratio, liver enzymes, Gallium scan (PPD, trichophyton, *Candida,* mumps streptodornase-streptokinase)

*PCR = Polymerase chain reaction

occasionally from the vitreous or retinal biopsy specimens during the acute phase of the disease. Polymerase chain reaction (PCR) may be helpful. Electronmicroscopy shows viral particles in tissue specimens.

D. **Subacute Sclerosing Panencephalitis**
1. **Clinical Findings:** Gradual mental deterioration with personality changes that precede the retinitis. Fundus examination shows focal retinitis involving the posterior pole in both eyes, and patients may develop optic atrophy.
2. **Laboratory Tests:** High rubeola antibody titers in serum and cerebrospinal fluid.

II. BACTERIAL INFECTIONS
A. **Tuberculosis**
1. **Clinical Findings:** Anterior granulomatous uveitis, mild to moderate vitritis, and multifocal choroiditis.
2. **Laboratory Tests:** Positive purified protein derivative, multifocal choroiditis may be seen in patients with miliary tuberculosis, chest radiograph may show active or healed lesions. Isolation of *Mycobacterium tuberculosis* from infected tissue specimens on Lowenstein-Jensen medium.

B. **Syphilis**
1. **Clinical Findings:** Granulomatous or nongranulomatous anterior uveitis, vitritis, retinitis, and multifocal choroiditis.
2. **Laboratory Tests:** Serum fluorescent treponemal antibody absorption test (FTA-ABS) and Veneral Disease Research Laboratory (VDRL) test.

C. **Nocardia Endophthalmitis**
1. **Clinical Findings:** Chronic lung disease; patients may have liver abscess. Ocular involvement may be unilateral or bilateral with minimal anterior segment involvement. Mild to moderate vitritis and multifocal choroidal infiltration with overlying retinitis. Retinal detachment may occur.

D. **Meningococcal Retinochoroiditis**
1. **Clinical Findings:** *Neisseria meningitidies* may cause juxtapapillary retino-

choroiditis in patients with meningitis. Patients may have multifocal retinitis and vitritis.
2. **Laboratory Tests:** Blood cultures, lumbar puncture, vitreous aspiration, and demonstration of organisms on culture and smears.

III. PARASITIC INFECTIONS
A. **Ocular Toxoplasmosis**
1. **Clinical Findings:** Yellow-white necrotizing retinitis with surrounding edema. Pigmented atrophic retinochoroiditic scar adjacent and contiguous to the lesion or elsewhere in the fundus. Vitreous cell strands or precipitates. Focal retinitis vasculitis may occur. Edema of the retina and hyperemia of the optic nerve may be observed with large granulomatous lesions of the posterior pole.
2. **Laboratory Tests:** Sabin-Feldman Dye test, indirect fluorescent antibody test, hemagglutination, or enzyme-linked immunosorbent assay (ELISA). Radiograph of the skull is helpful to confirm calcific deposits in patients with congenital toxoplasmosis. Tests for toxoplasma antigens or antibodies in ocular fluids may be performed. Polymerase chain reaction may be helpful.

B. **Toxocariasis**
1. **Clinical Findings:** Unilateral; in most cases marked inflammatory reaction in the eye with vitritis, peripheral focal whitish granuloma anywhere in the posterior pole or extending with whitish exudates and fibrosis toward the pars plana. Dragging of the retina or optic nerve head may occur. Patients may have moderate to severe vitritis.
2. **Laboratory Tests:** ELISA for *Toxocara canis* antibodies. Demonstration of eosinophils in vitreous specimens.

C. **Onchocerciasis**
1. **Ocular Findings:** Cutaneous skin nodules. The cornea may show nummular keratitis and sclerosing keratitis.

Anterior uveitis with microfilaria may be seen in the anterior chamber swimming actively like silver threads. Posterior uveitis may occur with focal retinitis and pigment proliferation. Areas of focal retinitis may occur with optic atrophy.

2. **Laboratory Tests:** Skin biopsy and microscopic examination looking for the live microfilaria.

D. Cysticercosis

1. **Clinical Findings:** Live larvae may be seen migrating under the retina. Death of the organism is associated with severe inflammatory reaction. This leads to chronic inflammatory reaction and retinochoroiditic scarring and retinal gliosis.

2. **Laboratory Tests:** Include radiograph of the skull, which may show multiple calcification.

IV. FUNGAL INFECTIONS

A. Candida Retinitis

1. **Clinical Findings:** Focal whitish elevated retinitis; string of pearls exudates may be seen. Vitreous shows evidence of cells with vitreous puffballs.

2. **Laboratory Tests:** Vitreous aspiration for smears and for isolation of *Candida* on Sabouraud's agar.

B. Cryptococcus

1. **Clinical Findings:** The disease may be associated with chronic cryptococcus meningitis. The ocular findings show anterior uveitis with vitreous cells and multifocal chorioretinitis.

2. **Laboratory Tests:** Include spinal fluid for examination for cryptococcal antigen titer or India ink preparation to demonstrate the *Cryptococcus neoformans.* Vitreous aspiration may be subjected to culture and cytology.

C. Histoplasmosis

1. **Clinical Findings:** Multifocal atrophic nummular choroidal scars, peripapillary atrophy, hemorrhagic disciform maculopathy with subretinal neovascularization. The vitreous shows no inflammatory cells.

2. **Laboratory Tests:** There is no specific diagnostic test. The diagnosis is made presumptively based on the clinical picture.

D. Aspergillosis

1. **Clinical Findings:** Usually occurs in patients who are immunologically suppressed. The clinical findings consist of vitritis with focal retinitis consisting of white elevated lesions.

2. **Laboratory Tests:** Should be performed, including blood cultures and vitreous aspiration.

V. AUTOIMMUNE DISEASES

A. Behcet's Disease

1. **Clinical Findings:** Definite Behcet's (complete type): all four major criteria of the disease are observed, including uveitis, skin lesions, genital ulcers, and oral ulcers. Probable Behcet's (incomplete type): ocular lesions with one other major criterion or three minor criteria. Clinical findings of posterior uveitis consist of vitreous cells, strands or opacities, retinal phlebitis, retinal hemorrhages, focal retinitis, papillitis, and systemic macular edema. Optic atrophy may occur in the late stages of the disease.

2. **Laboratory Tests:** Pathergy skin test, human leukocyte antigen (HLA) typing for HLA B51. Elevation of total immunoglobulins may be demonstrated in some patients during the activity of the disease.

B. Vogt-Koyanagi-Harada Syndrome

1. **Clinical Findings:** Patients present with prodromal symptoms of fever, headache, malaise, and nausea. Patients also may complain of headaches, neck stiffness, dysacousia tinnitus, loss of hair, vertigo, and hearing loss. The major clinical findings include anterior granulomatous uveitis or nongranulomatous uveitis, vitreous cells, exudative retinal detachment with areas of focal retinal pigment epitheliitis. In the after-math of the disease, patients show retinal pigment epithelial

migration and loss of the retinal pigment epithelium. Nonocular clinical findings include vitiligo, poliosis, alopecia, and hearing loss.

2. **Laboratory Tests:** Include disturbances in the audiogram, abnormal electroencephalogram. Cerebrospinal fluid shows increased protein and pleocytosis with predominance of lymphocytes. There is an association with HLA-DRB1*04 and HLA-DR4.

VI. DISEASES OF UNKNOWN CAUSES
A. Sarcoidosis
1. **Clinical Findings:** Lid or conjunctival granulomas, interstitial keratitis,

anterior granulomatous uveitis with Koeppe's and Busacca's nodules of the iris, vitreous exudation, retinal periphlebitis with candlewax drippings, and optic nerve granulomas.

2. **Laboratory Tests:** Chest radiograph may show bilateral hilar adenopathy. Serum lysozyme and angiotensin-converting enzyme are elevated (the tests are not specific for sarcoidosis). Lacrimal gland biopsy. Other laboratory tests include purified protein derivative, calcium, and total protein serum and Gallium scan.

B. Retinal Pigment Epitheliitis: Antibodies to Hepatitis C.

Fluorescein Angiography in Patients with Posterior Uveitis

Disease	Findings
1. Acute multifocal pigment placoid epitheliopathy	Lesions block fluorescence early or hypofluorescence of choriocapillaris. Late in the angiography the lesions stain.
2. Acute retinal necrosis	Leakage of the dye around the optic nerve head and segmental staining of blood vessels and vascular leakage. Localized retinal infiltrates block the dye early and stain late.
3. Behcet's disease	Staining of blood vessels. Leakage of retinal blood vessels. Neovascularization.
4. Birdshot retinochoriodopathy	Early hypofluorescence of lesions and late hyperfluorescence (active lesions) *Lesions may not be apparent on fluorescence angiogram.*
5. Cytomegalovirus retinitis	Leakage and stain of retinal blood vessels. Hyperfluorescence in areas of leakage *and in central part of lesion.* Brushfire-like retinitis stain late at edges. Hemorrhages block fluorescein.
6. Geographic choroiditis	Early blockage of dye at active advancing edge with late staining.
7. Histoplasmosis	Window-type defects with hyperfluorescence around optic nerve head. Subretinal macular neovascularization.
8. Intermediate uveitis	Cystoid macular edema. Leakage of dye and neovascularization in areas of optic nerve head.
9. Sarcoidosis	Early leakage of retinal blood vessels and late staining of vascular wall. Hyperfluorescence in areas of sarcoid granuloma.
10. Syphilis	Areas of blockage and window defects of retinal pigment epithelium (RPE). Choroidal neovascularization staining of optic nerve head in optic papillitis. Early leakage and late staining of retinal blood vessel wall in vasculitis. Patchy hyperfluorescence in cases with retinitis.
11. Toxoplasmosis	*Active lesions:* Hyperfluorescence of area of retinitis. Early leakage and late staining in vasculitis. Obliteration of dye in vascular occlusion. *Inactive lesions:* Areas of blockage of dye (pigment). Late staining of scars. *Sequalae:* Window defects. In punched-out lesions, bare sclera shows late stain, retinal vascularization, choroidal neovascularization, anteriovenous anastomoses.
12. Vogt-Koyanagi-Harada	Multiple areas of leakage from areas of focal inflammation in the choriocapillaris, giving rise to the typical Christmas tree appearance. Confluent areas of leakage and late staining of the optic nerve head may be seen. Subretinal neovascularization may occur.

QUESTIONAIRE FOR PATIENTS WITH POSTERIOR UVEITIS

Name: _____

Sex: _____

Birthdate: _____

Occupation: _____

This questionnaire is designed to obtain medical history from the patient before presenting to the examining ophthalmologist.

I. EARS, NOSE AND THROAT:

Do you complain of frequent severe headaches?...................... Yes No

Do you often have spells of dizziness? .... Yes No

Do you have numbness or tingling in any part of the body? ... Yes No

Have you ever had paralysis of any part of the body?.............. Yes No

Have you ever had convulsions or seizures?............................. Yes No

Have you ever had or sustained injury? .... Yes No

Have you had surgery on your mastoid? .... Yes No

Do you hear ringing or constant noises in your ears? .... Yes No

Have you had ear infection? .... Yes No

Have you had your tonsils or adenoids removed? .... Yes No

Have you had nosebleeds?........... Yes No

Have radiographs been taken of your sinuses? .... Yes No

Do you have frequent spells of sneezing?................................. Yes No

Have you had your teeth examined in the past year?............... Yes No

Have you had abscess of any tooth?.. Yes No

II. JOINTS AND BONES:

Have you had swelling of any joint in the body?..................... Yes No

Do you complain of frequent muscle aches?.......................... Yes No

Do you complain of pain in the back? .... Yes No

Do you have a stiff back in the morning? .... Yes No

Have you had redness or localized induration over the lower extremities (tibia)?................ Yes No

III. GENITOURINARY TRACT:

Have you ever had kidney, bladder, or urethral disease?........ Yes No

If yes, please explain.

_____

_____

Have ever passed blood in the urine?..................................... Yes No

Do you have burning on urination or discharge? .... Yes No

For males: Have you ever had discharge from the penis?..... Yes No

For females: Have you ever had vaginal discharge?................ Yes No

Have you ever had ulcers or skin lesions in the genital area? ... Yes No

IV. RESPIRATORY SYSTEM:

Have you had constant coughing?...................................... Yes No

Have you ever coughed up blood?................................... Yes No

Have you had any chronic chest disease?................................. Yes No

Did you live with anyone who had tuberculosis?.................. Yes No

Have you had severe sweat at night?..................................... Yes No

V. CARDIOVASCULAR SYSTEM:

Have you had heart problems?.. Yes No

Do you suffer from pain in the legs on walking?.................... Yes No

Have you had swelling of the legs?..................................... Yes No

Have you had difficulty breathing?...................................... Yes No

VI. GASTROINTESTINAL TRACT:

Have you suffered from frequent loose bowel movements? ..... Yes No

Have you had bloody diarrhea? Yes No

Have you had jaundice in the past?..................................... Yes No

Have you had any serious liver disease?................................. Yes No

VII. NERVOUS SYSTEM:

Have you had any neurologic problem?............................. Yes No

Have you had paresthesia, numbness, or paresis? .... Yes   No

Have you had frequent headaches? .... Yes   No

VIII. SOCIAL HISTORY:

State the names of the countries where you have lived in. _____

_____

_____

Are you taking any drug on a regular basis? .... Yes   No

If Yes, state the drug taken.

_____

Do you smoke? .... Yes   No

Do you consume smoked, undercooked, or raw meat? .... Yes   No

Do you have a pet at home? (birds, cats, dogs, etc.) .... Yes   No

If yes, what kind? _____

Do you have a sandbox for kittens at home?....................... Yes   No

Have you lived or do you live in areas of open wilderness? ... Yes   No

Do you consume unpasteurized milk or cheese? .... Yes   No

IX. MEDICAL HISTORY:

Have enjoyed good health in the past? .... Yes   No

Do you suffer from any chronic disease? .... Yes   No

If yes, please state._____

_____

Have you had any of the following conditions:

Cold sore? .... Yes   No
Tuberculosis?....................... Yes   No
Pneumonia?.......................... Yes   No
Rheumatism? .... Yes   No
Arthritis? .... Yes   No
Hay fever?........................... Yes   No
Asthma? .... Yes   No
Allergies?............................ Yes   No
Hives? .... Yes   No
Severe tonsillitis?............... Yes   No
Streptococcal infection?...... Yes   No
Diarrhea?............................. Yes   No
Severe influenza?............... Yes   No

Diabetes?............................. Yes   No
Skin rashes? .... Yes   No
Pleurisy? .... Yes   No
Parasitic infection?............... Yes   No
Fever? .... Yes   No
Anemia?............................... Yes   No
Syphilis? .... Yes   No
Cancer? .... Yes   No
Gonorrhea? .... Yes   No

Have you had bleeding from your nose, lungs, bowel or rectum?
.... Yes   No

Have you had treatment with radiation? .... Yes   No

Have you had any serious injury?
.... Yes   No

List types of operations you have had and their dates: _____

_____

_____

_____

Have you had any skin lesions in the past?............................. Yes   No

Have you had any skin ulcers in the past?............................. Yes   No

Have you had skin rash?............. Yes   No

X. FAMILY HISTORY:

Has anyone in your family (other than you) had tuberculosis, arthritis, severe anemia, high blood pressure, diabetes, allergies, hay fever, asthma, hives, gouts, syphilis, or brucellosis (Malta fever)? .... Yes   No

Has anyone in your family had medical troubles of the eyes, skin, lungs, intestine, kidneys, brain, or glands? .... Yes   No

XI. PRESENT ILLNESS:

What is your main complaint? _____

_____

What brought you to the doctor, and how long have you had this complaint? _____

_____

State your height and weight_____

_____

OPHTHALMIC ETYMOLOGIES

acinus	(Latin) grape	lentigo	(Latin) lens, lentis = lentil (pl: lentigines)
blepharitis	(Greek) blepharon = eyelid	macula	(Latin) macula = spot, stain
canities	(Latin) canus = gray- or white-haired, hoary	madarosis	(Greek) madao = to fall off (of hair)
cataract	(Greek) katarrhaktes = a downrushing, a waterfall	molluscum	(Latin) molluscus = soft
catarrh	(Greek) katarrhoos = a running down (kata = down; rhein = to flow)	monilia	(Latin) monile = necklace
		mycosis	(Greek) mykes = fungus, osis = condition
chalazion	(Greek) chalazion = small hailstone (pl: chalazia)	nummular	(Latin) nummulus = coin
		phlyctenule	(Greek) phlyktaina = blister
delle	(Dutch) delle = slight depression or dimple, pit (pl: dellen)	pinguecula	(Greek) pinguis = fat
		pterygium	(Greek) pterygion = wing
		poliosis	(Greek) polios = gray
druse	(German) druse = gland (pl: drusen)	sclera	(Greek) skleros = hard
		scleromalacia	(Greek) scleros = hard, malaika = softening
embryotoxon	(Greek) embryo = embryo toxon = bow, arc-shaped	synophrys	(Greek) syn = joined, ophrys = eyebrow
fovea	(Latin) fovea = pit, fossa, or cup	syphilis	(Greek) siphlos = crippled "Syphilis sive de Morbo Gallico" By Fracastoro (1530). "Syphilus" was the shepherd in the poem. Derived from the Greek syn = together, philein to love
glaucoma	(Greek) glaukoma: glaukos = a dull, gray-green gleam		
gonorrhea	(Greek) gonos = seed, offspring rhein = to flow		
herpes	(Greek) herpeton = a crawling or creeping thing		
hordeolum	(Latin) hordeolum = barleycorn	uva	bunch of grapes
		uvea	fruit of *Vitis vinifera*
hyphema	(Greek) hypo = under haima = blood	vernal	(Latin) vernalis = of the spring
hypopyon	(Greek) hypo = under pyon = pus	verruca	(Latin) verruca = wart
		virus	(Latin) virus = poison
iris	(Greek) iris = rainbow, halo	vitiligo	(Latin) vitiligo = blanched skin (pl: vitili-gines)
keratitis	(Greek) keras = horn		
keratoacanthoma	(Greek) kerato = horn-shaped, acantho = thorn, oma = tumor	vitelliform	(Latin) vitella = yolk
		vitreous	(Latin) vitreus = glassy
		xanthelasma	(Greek) xanthos = yellow, elasma = beaten metal plate
lens	(Latin) lens, lentis = lentil		

APPENDIX

Clinical Trials Supported by the National Eye Institute

Retina and Choroid

EFFICACY AND SAFETY OF INTRAOCULAR LENS IMPLANTATION IN UVEITIS

Principal Investigator: Marc D. de Smet, M.D.

Institutions: 1 Clinical Center–NIH

Purpose

- To evaluate the safety and efficacy of intraocular lens implantation in patients with severe uveitis over a followup period of a least 1 year.
- To compare the postoperative inflammation following the implantation of a standard intraocular lens or a heparin surface modified lens.
- To determine which of two types of lens surfaces leads to less complications in patients with uveitis.

Background

Patients with uveitis are at high risk for significant complications following cataract surgery with an intraocular lens implant. These complications can be related to the surgery itself or can result from the lens material that is being implanted into the eye. The postoperative inflammation is often more intense and prolonged in patients with uveitis and may lead to the formation of iris to lens adhesions and an increased amount of flare. By *in vivo* specular microscopy of the lens surface, fibroblastlike cells and multinucleated giant cells can be seen on the surface of all implanted lenses, but the number usually decreases rapidly within several weeks following surgery. In patients with uveitis, cell deposits tend to persist for a longer period of time and, on occasion, giant cells will coalesce to form membranes which can obstruct the central visual axis and require a YAG laser to remove them. These giant cells are an indication of poor lens tolerance and are evidence of a foreign body reaction.

Modification of the lens surface with a uniform layer of heparin has been suggested to provide a more biocompatible surface. The total amount of heparin bound to the surface of the lens is approximately 0.5 μg which corresponds to less than 0.1 USP unit of heparin. Preclinical studies have shown a reduction in the degree of postoperative complications as compared to unmodified lenses.

Several retrospective series have looked at the use of intraocular lenses in patients with uveitis. However, no prospective controlled study to date has evaluated the safety and efficacy of intraocular lenses in uveitis patients. Furthermore, the surface modified lenses have never been tried in this patient population. Thus, it is appropriate to conduct a randomized controlled clinical trial of lens implantation in patients with uveitis.

Description

Patients with a history of recurrent anterior or posterior uveitis and anterior segment manifestations of past uveitis (e.g., synechiae, chronic flare, old keratic precipitates) will be entered in this prospective, double-masked randomized study. Eighty patients with uveitis under control with or without medications for at least 3 months and in need of cataract surgery will be randomized to receive either a standard PMMA lens or one that has been surface modified with heparin. Patients will be officially entered into the study at the time of surgery, after the nucleus and cortex have been successfully removed by standard extracapsular extraction or by phacoemulsification. The patient will then be followed periodically for a minimum of 1 year. The use of antiinflammatory medications will be closely monitored. Ocular inflammation will be assessed by careful clinical examination and the use of laser photometry. The development of synechiae, lens decentration or lens capture by the iris will be carefully documented and photographed. Lens tolerance will be assessed by determining the number and persistence of cell deposits on the lens surface. These will be assessed by using indirect specular microscopy of the lens surface and by determining the cell density and type on the anterior lens surface using serial photographs. These pictures will be graded by an independent investigator who will remain masked to the implanted lens type. Corneal endothelial cell counts will also be performed prior to surgery and at the end of 1 year. Any recurrence of posterior pole pathology will be documented by clinical exam and, where appropriate, by fluorescein angiography.

Patient Eligibility

Men and women eligible for the study must be age 18 or older and have a cataract in need of surgery and a history of recurrent anterior or posterior uveitis which has been under control for at least 3 months. Patients can only receive steroids and /or cyclosporine at the time of surgery, and patients taking cytotoxic agents will have to discontinue their use prior to surgery. Other exclusion criteria include: monocular patients, corneal pathology which would preclude visualization of the implant, uncontrolled glaucoma, diabetes, and patients unable to be followed for at least 1 year.

Patient Recruitment Status

Ongoing. Recruitment began in January 1993.

Current Status of Study

Ongoing.

Results

None to date.

Publications

None.

Clinical Center

Marc D. de Smet, M.D.
Laboratory of Immunology
National Eye Institute
National Institutes of Health
Warren Grant Magnuson Clinical Center
Building 10, Room 10N112
Bethesda, Maryland 20892
Telephone: (301) 496-3123

ENDOPHTHALMITIS VITRECTOMY STUDY (EVS)

Study Chairman: Bernard H. Doft, M.D.

Institutions: 28 Clinical Centers
3 Resource Centers

Purpose

- To determine the role of initial pars plana vitrectomy in the management of postoperative bacterial endophthalmitis.
- To determine the role of intravenous antibiotics in the management of bacterial endophthalmitis.
- To determine which factors, other than treatment, are predictors of outcome in postoperative bacterial endophthalmitis.

Background

Endophthalmitis is a serious ocular infection that can result in blindness. Approximately 70 percent of cases occur as a direct complication of intraocular surgery. Current management requires culture of intraocular contents and intravitreal antibiotic administration. Vitrectomy surgery may be beneficial in the management of endophthalmitis by removing infecting organisms and their toxins and has been shown to be of value in various animal models of endophthalmitis. However, human studies have not shown an advantage to vitrectomy with intraocular antibiotics compared to intraocular antibiotics alone.

In all large comparison studies to date, eyes with the worst initial presentations were those selected for vitrectomy. Because of the selection bias involved in determining which cases received vitrectomy, existing clinical information on the efficacy of the procedure for treating endophthalmitis is inconclusive. Determining the role of initial vitrectomy and whether certain subgroups of patients may benefit, will help the clinician in the management of endophthalmitis.

In addition, although systemic antibiotics historically have been used in the management of endophthalmitis, there has been little evidence to support their efficacy, but many reports of toxic systemic effects. In view of this, the role of systemic antibiotics will be assessed in the management of endophthalmitis.

Description

Endophthalmitis Vitrectomy Study (EVS) patients are randomized to one of two standard treatment strategies for the management of bacterial endophthalmitis. Eyes receive either (1) initial pars plana vitrectomy with intravitreal antibiotics, followed by retap and reinjection at 36-60 hours for eyes doing poorly as defined in the study, or (2) initial anterior chamber and vitreous tap/biopsy with injection of intravitreal antibiotics, followed by vitrectomy and reinjection at 36-60 hours in eyes doing poorly. In addition, all eyes are randomized to either treatment or no treatment with intravenous antibiotics.

Study endpoints are visual acuity and clarity of ocular media, the latter assessed both clinically and photographically. Each patient's initial endpoint assessment occurs at 3 months, after which procedures to improve vision, such as late vitrectomy for nonclearing ocular media, may be performed. The final outcome assessment occurs at 9 months. Multiple centers are cooperating by enrolling 420 eyes during a proposed 42-month recruitment period.

Patient Eligibility

Men and women are eligible for entry into the EVS if they have clinical signs and symptoms of bacterial endophthalmitis in an eye that has had cataract surgery or lens implantation within 6 weeks of onset of infection. The involved eye must have either hypopyon or enough clouding of anterior chamber or vitreous media to obscure clear visualization of second-order arterioles, a cornea and anterior chamber in the involved eye clear enough to visualize some part of the iris, and a cornea clear enough to allow the possibility of pars plana vitrectomy. The eyes should also have a visual acuity of 20/50 or worse and light perception or better.

Patients are ineligible when the involved eye is known at the time of study entry to have had any preexisting eye disease that limited best-corrected visual acuity to 20/100 or worse prior to development of cataract, any intraocular surgery prior to presentation (except for cataract extraction or lens implantation), treatment for endophthalmitis prior to presenting at the study center, or any ocular

or systemic condition preventing randomization to any of the study groups.

Patient Recruitment Status

Recruitment began in February 1990.

Current Status of Study

Ongoing.

Results

None to date.

Publications

None.

Clinical Centers

California

Richard R. Ober, M.D.
Department of Ophthalmology
University of Southern California
450 San Pablo Street-DOH
4703 Los Angeles, California 90033
Telephone: (213) 342-6450

Lon S. Poliner, M.D.
4150 Regents Park Row, Suite 200
La Jolla, California 92037
Telephone: (619) 558-9666

District of Columbia

Howard P. Cupples, M.D.
Department of Ophthalmology, PHC7
Georgetown University Medical Center
3800 Reservoir Road, N.W.
Washington, D.C. 20007
Telephone: (202) 687-4755

Florida

Mark E. Hammer, M.D.
617 Lakeview Road, Suite B
Clearwater, Florida 34616
Telephone: (813) 875-6373

Robert Mames, M.D.
Hillis Miller Medical Center
Box J-284
Department of Ophthalmology
University of Florida College of Medicine
Gainesville, Florida 326104284
Telephone: (904) 392-3451

Scott E. Pautler, M.D.
Tampa Bay Vitreo Retinal Associates
4600 North Habana Avenue, Suite 3
Tampa, Florida 33614
Telephone: (813) 879-5795

Peter Reed Pavan, M.D.
Eye Institute
University of South Florida
12901 B. B. Downs Boulevard
Tampa, Florida 33612-9400
Telephone: (813) 974-3820

Georgia

Antonio Capone, Jr., M.D.
Emory Eye Center, 5th Floor
Emory University
1327 Clifton Road, N.E.
Atlanta, Georgia 30322
Telephone: (404) 248-3956

Illinois

Kirk H. Packo, M.D.
Illinois Retina Associates, S.C.
71 West 156th Street, Suite 400
Harvey, Illinois 60426
Telephone: (708) 596-8710

Kentucky

Charles C. Barr, M.D.
Department of Ophthalmology

Kentucky Lions Eye Research Institute
University of Louisville
301 East Muhammad Ali Boulevard
Louisville, Kentucky 40202
Telephone: (502) 588-5466

Maryland

Peter Campochiaro, M.D.
Wilmer Eye Institute
Maumenee 719
The Johns Hopkins Medical Institutions
600 North Wolfe Street
Baltimore, Maryland 21218-9277
Telephone: (410) 955-5106

Richard A. Garfinkel, M.D.
Retina Group of Washington
5454 Wisconsin Avenue, Suite 1540
Chevy Chase, Maryland 20815
Telephone: (301) 656-8100

Vinod Lakhanpal, M.D.
Eye Associates
University of Maryland
419 West Redwood Street
Baltimore, Maryland 21201
Telephone: (410) 328-5906

Massachusetts

Donald D'Amico, M.D.
Massachusetts Eye and Ear Infirmary
243 Charles Street
Boston, Massachusetts 02114
Telephone: (617) 573-3291

Michigan

Raymond R. Margherio, M.D.
Associated Retinal Consultants, P.C.
Royal Oak Center
3535 West Thirteen Mile Road, Suite 636
Royal Oak, Michigan 48073
Telephone: (313) 288-2280

Andrew K. Vine, M.D.
Kellogg Eye Center
University of Michigan

1000 Wall Street
Ann Arbor, Michigan 48105
Telephone: (313) 763-0482

Minnesota

Herbert L. Cantrill, M.D.
6363 France Avenue South, Suite 570
Edina, Minnesota 55435
Telephone: (612) 929-1131

Mark W. Balles, M.D.
Department of Ophthalmology
University of Minnesota
Box 493 UMHC, Room 9-240 PWB
516 Delaware Street, S.E.
Minneapolis, Minnesota 55455
Telephone: (612) 625-4400

New Jersey

David L. Yarian, M.D.
Retina-Vitreous Center, P.A.
Medi-Plex Suite 310
98 James Street
Edison, New Jersey 08820
Telephone: (908) 906-1887

Ohio

Robert B. Chambers, D.O.
Ohio State University
456 West 10th Avenue
Columbus, Ohio 43210
Telephone: (614) 293-8041

Phillip T. Nelsen, M.D.
Retina Consultants of NW Ohio
JOBST Tower, Suite E
2109 Hughes Drive
Toledo, Ohio 43606
Telephone: (419) 479-6180

Thomas A. Rice, M.D.
Retina Associates of Cleveland
26900 Cedar Road, Suite 303
Beachwood, Ohio 44122
Telephone: (216) 831-5700

Oklahoma

Reagan H. Bradford, Jr., M.D.
Dean A. McGee Eye Institute
University of Oklahoma
608 Stanton L.Young Boulevard
Oklahoma City, Oklahoma 73104
Telephone: (405) 271-7232

Pennsylvania

Bernard H. Doft, M.D.
Retina Vitreous Consultants
3501 Forbes Avenue, Suite 500
Pittsburgh, Pennsylvania 15213
Telephone: (412) 683-5300

Thomas Gardner, M.D.
Department of Ophthalmology
College of Medicine
The Pennsylvania State University
Hershey, Pennsylvania 17033
Telephone: (717) 531-8783

Gary C. Brown, M.D.
Retinovitreous Associates
910 East Willow Grove
Philadelphia, Pennsylvania 19118
Telephone: (215) 233-4300

Texas

H. Michael Lambert, M.D.
Alkek Eye Center
Smith Tower, Suite 1501
6550 Fannin Boulevard
Houston, Texas 77030
Telephone: (713) 798-6100

Wisconsin

Dennis P. Han, M.D.
Eye Institute
Milwaukee County Medical Complex
Medical College of Wisconsin
8700 West Wisconsin Avenue
Milwaukee, Wisconsin 53226
Telephone: (414) 257-5341

Resource Centers

Chairman's Office

Bernard H. Doft, M.D.
Retina-Vitreous Consultants
3501 Forbes Avenue, Suite 500
Pittsburgh, Pennsylvania 15213
Telephone: (412) 683-5300
Fax: (412) 621-4833

Coordinating Center

Sheryl F. Kelsey, Ph.D.
Department of Epidemiology
The University of Pittsburgh
127 Parran Hall
130 DeSoto Street
Pittsburgh, Pennsylvania 15261
Telephone: (412) 624-1607

Fundus Photograph Reading Center

Matthew D. Davis, M.D.
Department of Ophthalmology
University of Wisconsin
WARF Building, Room 417
610 North Walnut
Madison, Wisconsin 53705
Telephone: (608) 263-4538
Fax: (608) 263-4525

NEI Representative

Donald F. Everett, M.A.
National Eye Institute
Executive Plaza South, Suite 350
6120 Executive Boulevard
Rockville, Maryland 20892
Telephone: (301) 496-5983
Fax: (301) 402-0528

Data and Safety Monitoring Committee

Kathryn Davis, Ph.D., Chair
University of Washington
Seattle, WA

Stanley P. Azen, Ph.D.
University of Southern California
Los Angeles, CA

Preston Covey, Ph.D.
Carnegie Mellon University
Pittsburgh, PA

Brooks W. McCuen, M.D.
Duke University
Durham, NC 27710

Andrew Packer, M.D.
Consulting Ophthalmology, P.C.
Hartford, CT

Ex Officio Members

Matthew D. Davis, M.D.
University of Wisconsin
Madison, WI

Bernard H. Doft, M.D.
Retina-Vitreous Consultants
Pittsburgh, PA

Donald F. Everett, M.A.
National Eye Institute
Bethesda, MD

Sheryl F. Kelsey, Ph.D.
University of Pittsburgh
Pittsburgh, PA

EVALUATION OF THE EFFECT OF ANTIFLAMMIN ON ACUTE ANTERIOR UVEITIS

Principal Investigator: Chi-Chao Chan, M.D.

Institution: 1 Clinical Center

Purpose

To evaluate the effectiveness and toxicity of anti-flammin, a potent phospholipase A_2 (PLA_2) inhibitor, in the treatment of acute anterior uveitis.

Background

Anterior uveitis is the most common form of uveitis. A single episode of anterior uveitis (acute or active anterior uveitis) causes pain and photophobia, but rarely results in permanent visual loss. Usually, acute anterior uveitis runs a short course (less than 4 to 6 weeks duration) with a 10-20 percent chance of recurrence over many years. These recurrences can eventually induce secondary glaucoma and cataracts, causing visual loss. In order to relieve its symptoms, anterior uveitis is usually treated with topical corticosteroids and cycloplegics. However, adverse side effects from these drugs, such as cataract formation and glaucoma induction, are common with prolonged application. Thus, therapeutic agents with potent anti-inflammatory effects and without associated adverse side effects need to be investigated.

PLA$_2$ is an esterase that specifically hydrolyzes the Sn$_2$ ester bond in cell membrane glycerophospholipids and generates free fatty acids. When the fatty acid is arachidonic acid, this reaction initiates the well-known arachidonic acid cascade that acts through cycloxygenase and lipoxygenase to generate numerous inflammatory mediators such as prostaglandins and leukotrienes. PLA$_2$ is involved in a myriad of cellular processes including leukotaxis and platelet activation. Thus, PLA$_2$ inhibitor has a potent anti-inflammatory effect. Antiflammin is a synthetic oligopeptide derived from the region of the highest amino acid sequence similarity between uteroglobin and lipocortin I. It has potent PLA$_2$ inhibitory and anti-platelet activating factor activities *in vitro*. It also demonstrates antiinflammatory effects *in vivo* without the known side effects of corticosteroids. It has been demonstrated that topical antiflammin can suppress endotoxin-induced uveitis, an experimental model of acute anterior uveitis, in the Lewis rat. The potency is similar to topical corticosteroids, and no adverse side effects have been observed. Thus, this clinical trial will examine the effect of topical antiflammin on acute anterior uveitis.

Description

A total of 78 patients with an acute attack of unilateral or bilateral anterior uveitis are being recruited for this study. Participants will be randomized to receive antiflammin and cycloplegics or placebo and cycloplegics. Both the patient and physician will be masked to the randomization. One drop of antiflammin or placebo solution will be administered every 2 hours, for a total of seven times a day (while awake) for 2 weeks to the affected eye. During these 2 weeks, the patient will be examined every other day. The medication will then be tapered and the patient will not be seen until the next uveitis attack. Patient followup will be done by telephone every 4 months for a period of 2 years. If the anterior uveitis worsens, the patient will then be switched to topical corticosteroids.

Patient Eligibility

Men and women between the ages of 18 and 60 years with acute iridocyclitis, either idiopathic or associated with systemic disease (ankylosing spondylitis, Reiter's syndrome, etc.) will be entered into the study. Patients who have recurrent attacks also will be eligible as long as they have not yet been treated with any form of corticosteroid therapy for at least 3 days since the attack. Patients with the following conditions are not eligible: sight-threatening diseases such as glaucoma; posterior pole disease; infections; corneal pathology; post-traumatic iridocyclitis; and more than 180° synechiae. Pregnant or nursing women are also excluded. Patients will be evaluated for visual acuity, by slit lamp and Kowa flare cell meter for anterior chamber inflammation, intraocular pressure, pachymetry, and will have iris photography. Dilated fundus and lens examinations are also included.

Patient Recruitment Status

Ongoing. Recruitment began in December 1992.

Current Status of Study

Ongoing.

Results

None to date.

Publications

Chan CC, Ni M, Miele L, Cordella-Miele E, Ferrick M, Mukherjee AB, Nussenblatt RB: Effects of antiflammins on endotoxin-induced uveitis in rats. Arch Ophthalmol 1991;109:278–281.

Clinical Center

Chi-Chao Chan, M.D.
National Eye Institute
National Institutes of Health
Warren Grant Magnuson Clinical Center
Building 10, Room 10N202
Bethesda, MD 20892
Telephone: (301) 496-3123

GANCICLOVIR IMPLANT STUDY FOR CYTOMEGALOVIRUS RETINITIS

Principal Investigators: Daniel F. Martin, M.D., Rajiv Anand, M.D., and Robert B. Nussenblatt, M.D.

Institutions: 2 Clinical Centers
2 Resource Centers

Purpose

To determine the therapeutic efficacy of a sustained-release intraocular drug delivery system for ganciclovir therapy of cytomegalovirus (CMV) retinitis in patients with AIDS.

Background

CMV retinitis occurs in 20-30 percent of patients with AIDS and is the leading cause of visual loss in these patients. At present, ganciclovir and foscarnet are the only two drugs that have been approved by the Food and Drug Administration for the treatment of CMV retinitis. The therapeutic regimen for each drug consists of a 2-week induction period followed by daily maintenance intravenous infusions. Unfortunately, CMV retinitis usually progresses despite daily maintenance therapy, and both drugs are associated with significant systemic toxicity that often limits their therapeutic usefulness. As an alternative to intravenous administration, direct intravitreal injections of ganciclovir have been studied and have been shown to be effective in delaying the progression of CMV retinitis. The short half-life of the drug, however, necessitates one to two intraocular injections a week to maintain therapeutic levels. Widespread adoption of this technique has been limited due to the logistical difficulties and inherent risks associated with numerous intravitreal injections.

A drug delivery system capable of continuous delivery of ganciclovir into the vitreous cavity has recently been developed. The device consists of a 6-mg pellet of ganciclovir that is coated with a series of polymers with variable permeability to ganciclovir. The device is surgically implanted through the pars plana. At present, two devices are under study: one that releases ganciclovir at a rate of 2 μg/hr and another that releases ganciclovir at a rate of 1 μg/hr. Results from phase I studies have been encouraging. The purpose of this study is to determine the therapeutic efficacy of each of the devices in a randomized, controlled clinical trial.

Description

Approximately 45 patients will be enrolled. All patients must have non-sight-threatening CMV retinitis ($>$ 3,000 μm from fovea and $>$ 1,500 μm from the optic disc) and not have been previously treated with ganciclovir or foscarnet. Patients with unilateral non-sight-threatening CMV retinitis will be randomly assigned to one of three groups: (1) immediate therapy with a device designed to release ganciclovir into the vitreous cavity at a rate of 2 μg/hr over approximately a 4-month period, (2) immediate therapy with a device designed to release ganciclovir into the vitreous cavity at a rate of 1 μg/hr over approximately an 8-month period, or (3) delayed therapy. In patients with bilateral non-sight-threatening CMV retinitis, one eye will be randomly assigned to receive a ganciclovir implant with the other eye assigned to deferral. The eye assigned to immediate treatment will be further randomized to receive either a 2 μg/hr or 1 μg/hr device.

The primary endpoint will be time to retinitis progression, defined as the time (days) from initiating therapy until advancement of 750 μm over a 750 gum front of any border of any lesion is observed. Standardized nine field photographs will be taken at 2-week intervals and analyzed in a masked fashion by the Fundus Photograph Reading Center to determine evidence of CMV retinitis progression.

Patient Eligibility

All patients must have AIDS as defined by the Centers for Disease Control and non-sight-threatening CMV retinitis (> 3,000 μm from the fovea and > 1,500 μm from the optic disc). Patients cannot have been previously treated with systemic ganciclovir or foscarnet and must not have evidence of other organ involvement with CMV. Patients must have an absolute neutrophil count (ANC) greater than 1,000 cells/ml and a platelet count greater than 25,000/mm³.

Patient Recruitment Status

Ongoing. Recruitment began November 1992.

Current Status of Study

Ongoing.

Results

None to date.

Publications

None.

Clinical Centers

Maryland

Daniel F. Martin, M.D.
Robert B. Nussenblatt, M.D.
National Eye Institute
National Institutes of Health

Warren Grant Magnuson Clinical Center Building 10, Room 10N202
Bethesda, Maryland 20892
Telephone: (301) 496-3123

Texas

Rajiv Anand, M.D.
Department of Ophthalmology
University of Texas Southwestern Medical Center
5323 Harry Hines Boulevard
Dallas, Texas 75235-9057

Resource Centers

Chairmen's Office

Daniel F. Martin, M.D.
Robert B. Nussenblatt, M.D.
National Eye Institute
National Institutes of Health
Warren Grant Magnuson Clinical Center
Building 10, Room 10N202
Bethesda, Maryland 20892
Telephone: (301) 496-3123

Fundus Photograph Reading Center

Matthew D. Davis, M.D.
Department of Ophthalmology
University of Wisconsin
610 North Walnut Street, Room 417
Madison, Wisconsin 53705-5240
Telephone: (608) 263-6071

Data and Safety Monitoring Committee

Susan Ellenberg, Ph.D.
Food and Drug Administration
Rockville, MD

Frederick L. Ferris III, M.D.
National Eye Institute
Bethesda, MD

Douglas A. Jabs, M.D.
The Johns Hopkins University
Baltimore, MD

Marvin Podgor, Ph.D.
National Eye Institute
Bethesda, MD

Ex Officio Members

Wiley A. Chambers, M.D.
Food and Drug Administration
Rockville, MD

Emily Y. Chew, M.D.
National Eye Institute
Bethesda, MD

Robert B. Nussenblatt, M.D.
National Eye Institute
Bethesda, MD

MACULAR PHOTOCOAGULATION STUDY (MPS)

Study Chairman: Stuart L. Fine, M.D.

Institutions: 15 Clinical Centers
3 Resource Centers

Purpose

To evaluate laser treatment of choroidal neovascularization (CNV) through randomized, controlled clinical trials. The Macular Photocoagulation Study (MPS) currently consists of three sets of randomized controlled clinical trials. Change in best-corrected visual acuity from baseline is the primary outcome for all MPS trials. Other measures of vision are evaluated in each set of trials. The purpose of each is described below.

Argon Study: To determine whether argon blue-green laser photocoagulation of leaking abnormal blood vessels in choroidal neovascular membranes outside the fovea [200 to 2,500 microns from the center of the foveal avascular zone (FAZ)] is of benefit in preventing or delaying loss of central vi-

sion in patients with age-related (senile) macular degeneration (AMD), presumed ocular histoplasmosis (POH), and idiopathic neovascular membranes (INVM). A separate trial was conducted for each of the three underlying conditions.

Krypton Study: To determine whether krypton red laser photocoagulation of choroidal neovascular lesions with the posterior border 1 to 199 microns from the center of the FAZ is of benefit in preventing or delaying large losses of visual acuity in patients with AMD, POH, and INVM. A separate trial was conducted for each of the three underlying conditions.

Foveal Study: To determine whether laser photocoagulation is of benefit in preventing or delaying further visual acuity loss in patients with new (never treated) or recurrent (previously treated) choroidal neovascularization under the center of the FAZ. Two separate trials, one for each type of lesion, are underway.

Background

Age-related macular degeneration is the leading cause of severe visual acuity loss in the United States among people over age 60. Presumed ocular histoplasmosis is a leading cause of visual loss in young and middle-aged persons living in the "histo" belt, an area that includes all of Arkansas, Kentucky, Missouri, Tennessee, and West Virginia and major portions of Alabama, Illinois, Indiana, Iowa, Kansas, Louisiana, Maryland, Mississippi, Nebraska, Ohio, Oklahoma, Texas, and Virginia. Both disorders are associated with CNV that damages the macula. Idiopathic CNV leads to acute loss of central vision but is not attributed to any known disease process. In all three disorders, visual loss results from complications of CNV in the macula.

Description

The first set of MPS randomized trials, the Argon Study, focused on the effectiveness of photocoagulation with argon blue-green laser in eyes with discrete extrafoveal neovascular membranes. The study investigators began recruiting patients in 1979. It was estimated that 550 patients with AMD and 750 with POH would be required. Followup was to continue for 5 years to determine whether argon laser photocoagulation treatment could prevent or delay visual acuity loss in these patients.

After the initiation of the Argon Study, a new krypton red laser became available. The new wavelength offered theoretical advantages over the argon laser for treating CNV that extended inside the FAZ of the macula. Availability of the new laser led to an expansion of the MPS. The Krypton Study design was analogous to the Argon Study, with the investigation of three underlying conditions, except that lesions were closer to the FAZ center.

The third set of MPS clinical trials, the Foveal Study, was designed to determine whether laser photocoagulation is effective for delaying or preventing further visual acuity loss in AMD patients who have subfoveal CNV. In the Foveal Study, argon green laser treatment has been compared with krypton red laser treatment of these lesions. It was originally projected that about 350 patients would be required for each clinical trial of the Foveal Study.

Patient Eligibility

Common Eligibility Criteria for the Argon, Krypton, and Foveal Studies: Eligible men and women must have been experiencing visual symptoms attributable to the macular lesion, such as decreased visual acuity or Amsler grid distortion, at the time of entry into the study and had visible hyperfluorescence characteristic of choroidal neovascularization on fluorescein angiography. AMD patients were 50 years of age or older and had drusen visible in the macula of at least one eye. POH patients were at least 18 years old and had at least one atrophic histo spot in one or both eyes. INVM patients were at least 18 years old and had no evidence of AMD, POH, angioid streaks, high myopia, diabetic retinopathy, or any other condition that could be presumed to be the cause of the neovascular membrane. In particular, INVM patients had neither drusen greater than MPS Standard Photograph No.1.1 nor histo spots in either eye.

Additional Patient Eligibility Criteria for the Argon Study: Each man or woman had a visible serous detachment of the sensory retina with a dif-

fuse area of leakage, a choroidal neovascular membrane outside the fovea (200 2,500 microns from the center of the FAZ), and visual acuity of 20/100 or better in the study eye.

Additional Patient Eligibility Criteria for the Krypton Study: All men and women had a neovascular lesion consisting of neovascularization, and possibly blood and/or pigment, that extended as close as 1 to 199 microns from the center of the FAZ. Visual acuity of the study eye was 20/400 or better.

Additional Patient Eligibility Criteria for the Foveal Study: Only men and women with AMD were eligible for this study. Fluorescein angiography of the eligible eye had to show evidence of a leaking choroidal neovascular membrane, some part of which extended under the center of the FAZ, or a neovascular lesion consisting of an old treatment scar and contiguous leaking neovascularization within 150 microns of the center of the FAZ. New, never-treated subfoveal lesions were less than 4 disc areas in size. Recurrent lesions were less than 6 disc areas in size, including the old treatment and new neovascularization. Best-corrected visual acuity was no better than 20/40 and no worse than 20/320.

Patient Recruitment Status

Recruitment for the MPS trials of laser treatment of extrafoveal neovascular lesions began in February 1979, for juxtafoveal CNV in January 1981, and for subfoveal CNV in February 1986. Recruitment was completed for the Argon Study in 1983, for the Krypton Study in 1987, and for the studies of new and recurrent subfoveal CNV in 1990.

Current Status of Study

Foveal Study: ongoing. Argon Study and Krypton Study: analysis and reporting.

Results

Recruitment of AMD patients in the Argon Study was halted in March 1982 and of POH and INVM patients in May 1983 after 236 patients with AMD, 262 with POH, and 67 with INVM had been enrolled. These decisions were based on findings that argon laser treatment, as applied in the study, can dramatically reduce severe visual acuity loss in these conditions. Patients in the Argon Study trials were discharged from the study as they completed 5 years of regular followup examinations.

In the Krypton Study, patient recruitment was halted for the POH trial in December 1986 because of evidence of treatment benefit in these patients. Recruitment of patients with AMD or INVM was halted in December 1987. In 1989, sufficient data had accumulated to demonstrate that there was a beneficial effect of krypton red laser treatment in eyes with AMD. The benefit was most pronounced in normotensive patients and disappeared among hypertensive patients. Findings for patients with INVM were intermediate between those of patients with AMD and POH. Patients in the Krypton Study were discharged as they completed 5 years of regular followup except for those enrolled during the last 2 years of patient accrual. All patients had been discharged from the study by March 31, 1991.

In December 1989, patient enrollment was completed in the Foveal Study trial for never-treated subfoveal choroidal neovascularization; 373 patients were randomized. Enrollment of patients with subfoveal recurrence after laser treatment continued until December 1990. Findings showing treatment benefit for both groups of eyes were published in September 1991. Patients have been discharged as they completed 4 years of followup. Those remaining will be discharged by December 1993.

Publications

Macular Photocoagulation Study Group: Argon laser photocoagulation for senile macular degeneration: Results of a randomized clinical trial. Arch Ophthalmol 1982;100: 912–918.

Macular Photocoagulation Study Group: Argon laser photocoagulation for ocular histoplasmosis: Results of a randomized clinical trial. Arch Ophthalmol 1982;100:912–918.

Macular Photocoagulation Study Group: Argon laser photocoagulation for idiopathic neovascularization: Results of a randomized clinical trial. Arch Ophthalmol 1983;101: 1358–1361.

Macular Photocoagulation Study Group: Changing the protocol: A case report from the Macular Photocoagulation Study. Controlled Clin Trials 1984;5:203–216.

Fine SL, Macular Photocoagulation Study Group: Early detection of extrafoveal neovascular membranes by daily central field evaluation. Ophthalmology 1985;92:603–609.

Macular Photocoagulation Study Group: Recurrent choroidal neovascularization after argon laser treatment for neovascular maculopathy. Arch Ophthalmol 1986,104:503–512.

Macular Photocoagulation Study Group: Argon laser photocoagulation for neovascular maculopathy. Three-year results from randomized clinical trials. Arch Ophthalmol 1986;104: 694–701.

Hillis A, Maguire M, Hawkins BS, Newhouse MM: The Markov process as a general method for nonparametric analysis of right-censored medical data. J Chron Dis 1986;39:595–604.

Macular Photocoagulation Study Group: Krypton laser photocoagulation for neovascular lesions of ocular histoplasmosis: Results of a randomized clinical trial. Arch Ophthalmol 1987;105:1499–1507.

Macular Photocoagulation Study Group: Persistent and recurrent neovascularization after krypton laser photocoagulation for neovascular lesions of ocular histoplasmosis. Arch Ophthalmol 1989;107:344–352.

Blackhurst DW, Maguire MG: Macular Photocoagulation Study Group: Reproducibility of refraction and visual acuity measurement under a standard protocol. Retina 1989;9(3): 163–169.

Chamberlin JA, Bressler NM, Bressler SB, Elman MJ, Murphy RP, Flood TP, Hawkins BS, Maguire MG, Fine SL: Macular Photocoagulation Study Group: The use of fundus photographs and fluorescein angiograms in the identification and treatment of choroidal neovascularization in the Macular Photocoagulation Study. Ophthalmology 1989;96(10): 1526–1534.

Macular Photocoagulation Study Group: Krypton laser photocoagulation for neovascular lesions of age-related macular degeneration. Results of a randomized clinical trial. Arch Ophthalmol 1990;108:816–824.

Macular Photocoagulation Study Group: Persistent and recurrent neovascularization after krypton laser photocoagulation for neovascular lesions of age-related macular degeneration. Arch Ophthalmol 1990;108:825–831.

Macular Photocoagulation Study Group: Krypton laser photocoagulation for idiopathic neovascular lesions. Results of a randomized clinical trial. Arch Ophthalmol 1990;108: 832–837.

Bressler SB, Maguire MG, Bressler NM, Fine SL: Macular Photocoagulation Study Group: Relationship of drusen and abnormalities of the retinal pigment epithelium to the prognosis of neovascular macular degeneration. Arch Ophthalmol 1990;108:1442–1447.

Hawkins BS, Prior MJ, Fisher MR, Blackhurst DW: Relationship between rate of patient enrollment and quality of clinical center performance in two multicenter trials in ophthalmology. Controlled Clin Trials 1990;11:374–394.

Bressler NM, Bressler SB, Alexander J, Javornik N, Fine SL, Murphy RP: Macular Photocoagulation Study Reading Center: Loculated fluid: A previously undescribed fluorescein angiographic finding in choroidal neovascularization associated with macular degeneration. Arch Ophthalmol 1991;109: 211–215.

Macular Photocoagulation Study Group: Argon laser photocoagulation for neovascular maculopathy. Five-year results from randomized clinical trials. Arch Ophthalmol 1991;109: 1109–1114.

Macular Photocoagulation Study Group: Laser photocoagulation of subfoveal neovascular lesions in age-related macular degeneration. Results of a randomized clinical trial. Arch Ophthalmol 1991;109:1219–1230.

Macular Photocoagulation Study Group: Laser photocoagulation of subfoveal recurrent neovascular lesions in age-related macular degeneration. Results of a randomized clinical trial. Arch Ophthalmol 1991;109:1232–1241.

Macular Photocoagulation Study Group: Subfoveal neovascular lesions in age-related macular degeneration. Guidelines for evaluation and treatment in the Macular Photocoagulation Study. Arch Ophthalmol 1991;109:1242–1257.

Orr PR, Blackhurst DW, Hawkins BS: Patient and clinic factors predictive of missed visits and inactive status in a multicenter clinical trial. Controlled Clin Trials 1991;13: 40–49.

Macular Photocoagulation Study Group: Five-year followup of fellow eyes of patients with age-related macular degeneration and unilateral extrafoveal choroidal neovascularization. Arch Ophthalmol (in press).

Clinical Centers

Florida

J. Donald M. Gass, M.D.
Bascom Palmer Eye Institute
University of Miami School of Medicine
900 N.W. 17th Street
Miami, Florida 33136
Telephone: (305) 326-6198

Georgia

Paul Sternberg, Jr., M.D.
Department of Ophthalmology
Emory Eye Center, Retina Service 4th Floor
Emory University
1327 Clifton Road, N.E.
Atlanta, Georgia 30322
Telephone: (404) 248-4120

Illinois

David H. Orth, M.D.
Illinois Retina Associates, S.C.
Vascular Services Department
Ingalls Memorial Hospital
Professional Office Building, Suite 400
One Ingalls Drive
Harvey, Illinois 60426
Telephone: (708) 596-8710, (708) 726-4949

Iowa

James C. Folk, M.D.
Department of Ophthalmology
University of Iowa
University Hospitals
Iowa City, Iowa 52242
Telephone: (319) 356-4338

Louisiana

Kurt A. Gitter, M.D.
Touro Medical Office Building
3525 Prytania Street, Suite 320
New Orleans, Louisiana 70115
Telephone: (504) 895-3961

Maryland

Neil M. Bressler, M.D.
Wilmer Ophthalmological Institute
The Johns Hopkins Medical Institutions
Maumenee Building, Room 21S
600 North Wolfe Street
Baltimore, Maryland 21287
Telephone: (301) 955-8343

Michigan

Raymond R. Margherio, M.D.
William Beaumont Hospital
Associated Retinal Consultants, P.C.
Beaumont Medical Building, Suite 632
3535 West Thirteen Mile Road
Royal Oak, Michigan 48072
Telephone: (313) 288-2280

Missouri

Dean B. Burgess, M.D.
Retina Consultants, Ltd.
East Pavilion Building, Suite 17413
One Barnes Hospital Plaza
St. Louis, Missouri 63110
Telephone: (314) 367-1181

Ohio

Lawrence J. Singerman, M.D.
Retina Associates of Cleveland
Mt. Sinai Medical Building
26900 Cedar Road, Room 303
Beachwood, Ohio 44122
Telephone: (216) 831-5700, (216) 221-2878

Oklahoma

C. P. Wilkinson, M.D.
McGee Eye Institute (A participating center until July 1991)
608 Stanton Young Drive
Oklahoma City, Oklahoma 73104
Telephone: (405) 271-6237

Oregon

Michael L. Klein, M.D.
Department of Ophthalmology
Oregon Health Sciences Center
3181 S.W. Sam Jackson Park Road
Portland, Oregon 97201
Telephone: (503) 494-7891

Texas

Gary E. Fish, M.D.
Texas Retina Associates
7150 Greenville Avenue, Suite 3400
Dallas, Texas 75231
Telephone: (214) 692-6941

Charles A. Garcia, M.D.
Hermann Eye Center
University of Texas Medical School

6411 Fannin Boulevard, MSB 7.226
Houston, Texas 77030
Telephone: (713) 792-7678

Wisconsin

Suresh R. Chandras M.D.
Department of Ophthalmology
Clinical Sciences Center
University of Wisconsin-Madison
600 Highland Avenue, F4/334
Madison, Wisconsin 53792
Telephone: (608) 263-4644

Thomas B. Burton, M.D.
Eye Institute, 2nd Floor
Milwaukee County Medical Complex
Medical College of Wisconsin
8700 West Wisconsin Avenue
Milwaukee, Wisconsin 53226
Telephone: (414) 257-5350

Resource Centers

Chairman's Office

Stuart L. Fine, M.D.
Scheie Eye Institute
University of Pennsylvania
51 North 39th Street
Philadelphia, Pennsylvania 19104
Telephone: (215) 662-9679

Coordinating Center

Barbara S. Hawkins, Ph.D.
Clinical Trials and Biometry
Wilmer Ophthalmological Institute
The Johns Hopkins Medical Institutions
550 North Broadway, 9th Floor
Baltimore, Maryland 21205
Telephone: (410) 955-8318

Reading Center

Neil M. Bressler, M.D.
Clinical Trials and Biometry
Wilmer Ophthalmological Institute

The Johns Hopkins Medical Institutions
550 North Broadway, 9th Floor
Baltimore, Maryland 21287
Telephone: (410) 955-8109

NEI Representative

Jack A. McLaughlin, Ph.D.
National Eye Institute
Executive Plaza South, Suite 350
6120 Executive Boulevard
Rockville, Maryland 20892
Telephone: (301) 496-5983

Data and Safety Monitoring Committee

Curtis L. Meinert, Ph.D., Chair
Johns Hopkins University
Baltimore, MD

Patricia McCormick Beamer
Summit, NJ

Argye Hillis, Ph.D.
Scott & White Memorial Hospital
Temple, TX

Lee M. Jampol, M.D.
Northwestern University Medical School
Chicago, IL

Edward B. McLean, M.D.
Seattle, WA

Bernard Rosner, Ph.D.
Harvard Medical School
Boston, MA

Barbara Safriet, L.L.M., J.D.
Yale University School of Law
New Haven, CT

Ex Officio Members

Stuart L. Fine, M.D.
Scheie Eye Institute
Philadelphia, PA

Barbara S. Hawkins, Ph.D.
Johns Hopkins University
Baltimore, MD

Maureen G. Maguire, Ph.D.
Johns Hopkins University
Baltimore, MD

Jack A. McLaughlin, Ph.D.
National Eye Institute
Bethesda, MD

M. Marvin Newhouse
Johns Hopkins University
Baltimore, MD

RANDOMIZED TRIAL OF ACETAZOLAMIDE FOR UVEITIS-ASSOCIATED CYSTOID MACULAR EDEMA

Principal Investigator: Scott M. Whitcup, M.D.

Institution: 1 Clinical Center–NIH

Purpose

To test the efficacy of acetazolamide for the treatment of uveitis-associated cystoid macular edema.

Background

Uveitis, an intraocular inflammatory disease, is the cause of about 10 percent of visual impairment in the United States. Uveitis may lead to many sight-threatening conditions including cataract, vitreal opacities, glaucoma, and, most commonly, cystoid macular edema. Reduction of swelling or edema within the retina is dependent on the movement of fluid from the retina through the choroid. A number of studies indicate that this process requires active transport of fluid ions by the retinal pigment epithelium, and may involve the carbonic anhydrase system. Current treatment of uveitis-associated cystoid macular edema requires the use of immunosuppressive or anti-inflammatory agents. However, many patients are either resistant or intolerant to this therapy. Recent reports suggest that acetazolamide, a carbonic anhydrose inhibitor that is used to lower intraocular pressure in some glaucoma patients, may be safe and effective in reducing uveitis-associated cystoid macular edema.

Description

Because the course of ocular inflammatory disease can be variable, a double-masked, randomized, cross-over trial has been designed to test the efficacy of acetazolamide compared to a placebo for the treatment of uveitis-associated cystoid macular edema. Randomized adult patients will receive either oral acetazolamide sodium 500 mg or a matched placebo every 12 hours for the first 4 weeks of the study. Children 8 years of age or older will receive a lesser dose. Following a 4-week period, during which no medication is given, patients will then receive a 4-week course of the opposite medication. Primary endpoints include reduction in cystoid macular edema as graded on fluorescein angiography and improvement in visual acuity as measured on standardized Early Treatment of Diabetic Retinopathy Study (ETDRS) charts. Laser acuity will also be assessed as a secondary outcome variable. Adverse effects of the acetazolamide therapy will be monitored by clinical and laboratory examinations.

A total of 40 patients will be recruited for the study. Patients will be seen at the beginning of the study for baseline measurements and at 4, 8, and 12 weeks after enrollment into the study.

Patient Eligibility

Males and females 8 years of age or older and weighing at least 35 kg (77 pounds) are eligible for the study. Patients must have a best corrected visual acuity of 20/40 or worse in at least one eye with cystoid macular edema demonstrable on fluorescein angiography.

Patients may be receiving systemic therapy for their uveitis. Exclusion criteria include: current use of acetazolamide as part of a therapeutic regimen; a history of hypersensitivity reactions to acetazolamide, sulfonamides, or angiography dye; unclear ocular media that would obscure fluorescein angiography; macular subretinal neovascularization or a macular hole; or inability to take acetazolamide for medical reasons.

Patient Recruitment Status

Ongoing. Recruitment began December 1990.

Current Status of Study

Ongoing.

Results

None to date.

Publications

None.

Clinical Center

Scott M. Whitcup, M.D.
National Eye Institute
National Institutes of Health
Warren Grant Magnuson Clinical Center
Building 10, Room 10N202
Bethesda, Maryland 20892
Telephone: (301) 496-3123

STUDIES OF THE OCULAR COMPLICATIONS OF AIDS (SOCA): CMV RETINITIS RETREATMENT TRIAL (CRRT)

Study Chairman: Douglas A. Jabs, M.D.

Institutions: 11 Clinical Centers
4 Resource Centers

Purpose

In order to address issues related to eye involvement in patients with the acquired immune deficiency syndrome (AIDS), the National Eye Institute has funded the Studies of Ocular Complications of AIDS (SOCA), a multicenter clinical trials group. SOCA's major activities involve evaluating treatments and treatment strategies for cytomegalovirus (CMV) retinitis, the most frequent ocular opportunistic infection in patients with AIDS. SOCA's initial clinical trial, the Foscarnet-Ganciclovir Cytomegalovirus Retinitis Trial (FGCRT) was completed in October 1992. SOCA's current trial is the CMV Retinitis Retreatment Trial (CRRT).

The purpose of the CMV Retinitis Retreatment Trial (CRRT) is:

- To compare the relative merits of three therapeutic regimens in patients with AIDS and CMV retinitis, who have been previously treated but whose retinitis is either nonresponsive or has relapsed. These three therapeutic regimens are: 1) foscarnet; 2) high-dose ganciclovir; and 3) combination foscarnet and ganciclovir.
- To compare two treatment strategies in patients with relapsed or nonresponsive CMV retinitis: 1) continuing with the same anti-CMV drug; or 2) switching to the alternate drug.

Background

CMV retinitis is the most common intraocular infection in patients with AIDS, affecting an estimated 20 percent to 25 percent of patients. Untreated, CMV retinitis is a progressive disorder, the end result of which is total retinal destruction and blindness. Given current projections for the AIDS epidemic, it is estimated that there may be as many as 30,000 to 50,000 patients with CMV retinitis in the United States in 1993.

Two drugs are now approved by the United States Food and Drug Administration for the treatment of CMV retinitis: ganciclovir (Cytovene®) and foscarnet (Foscavir®). Both drugs are currently approved only as an intravenous (IV) formulation. Each drug is given in a similar fashion, consisting of an initial 2-week high-dose treatment (induction), followed by long-term lower-dose (maintenance) treatment. All patients with CMV retinitis relapse when anti-CMV therapy is discontinued, generally within 2 to 3 weeks; therefore, maintenance therapy is required.

Despite the use of continuous maintenance therapy, maintenance therapy eventually relapse. Furthermore, the time to relapse progressively shortens with each successive relapse. While relapse can often be controlled by reinduction with the same drug followed by continued maintenance therapy, with each relapse, additional retina is destroyed. Therefore, treatment strategies designed to prolong the time to relapse are needed.

Current therapy with foscarnet is to begin with an induction dose of 60 mg/kg every 8 hours followed by a maintenance dose of 90 mg/kg/day. After the first relapse, the maintenance dose of foscarnet is generally increased to 120 mg/kg/day. Conversely, current practice for patients on ganciclovir is to use an induction of 5 mg/kg every 12 hours and maintenance dose of 5 mg/kg/day for each induction and maintenance course, whether or not there has been a previous relapse. One of the regimens to be tested in the CRRT is higher maintenance dose ganciclovir, 10 mg/kg/day. Pilot data from small, uncontrolled case series have suggested that combination therapy with both ganciclovir and foscarnet may be effective in controlling rapidly relapsing CMV retinitis, when therapy with a single agent alone has not been effective. Therefore, combination therapy will also be evaluated. Finally, because of a potential beneficial effect on the development of resistant CMV for patients with relapsed retinitis, it may be that switching to the alternate drug will significantly prolong the time to relapse.

Description

Approximately 300 patients will be enrolled in the CRRT. Eligible patients will have AIDS, CMV retinitis, have been previously treated for their retinitis with either ganciclovir or foscarnet, and have active disease despite previous therapy (nonresponsive or relapsed). Patients will be randomized to one of three treatments: (1) foscarnet; (2) high-dose ganciclovir; or (3) combination ganciclovir and foscarnet. Randomization will be stratified for prior drug therapy.

Patients randomized to the foscarnet arm will receive induction foscarnet at a dosage of 90 mg/kg every 12 hours for 2 weeks, followed by maintenance foscarnet at a dose of 120 mg/kg/day.

Patients randomized to high-dose ganciclovir will receive induction ganciclovir at a dosage of 5 mg/kg every 12 hours for 2 weeks, followed by maintenance ganciclovir at a dosage of 10 mg/kg/day. Patients randomized to the combination arm will continue on standard maintenance therapy with the drug they currently receive (either ganciclovir or foscarnet) and receive induction therapy with the other drug at standard doses, followed by maintenance therapy with both ganciclovir at 5 mg/kg/day and foscarnet at 90 mg/kg/day. Patients who relapse while on the assigned therapy will be reinduced and treated according to standardized treatment algorithms.

Because of the differences in drug administration methods, treatment will not be masked. However, evaluation of retinitis progression will be performed in a masked fashion by the Fundus Photograph Reading Center. Outcome measures of this trial include survival, retinitis progression, changes in visual function (visual acuity and visual fields), drug toxicity, and quality of life. Patients will be followed until death or common study closeout.

Patient Eligibility

Males and females eligible for the CRRT must be age 18 years or older and have AIDS and CMV retinitis. They must have active CMV despite a minimum of 28 days of previous treatment with an anti-CMV drug. Furthermore, they must have an absolute neutrophil count ≥ 500 cells/μl, platelet count $> 20,G00$ cells/μl, and a serum creatinine < 2.5 mg/dl in order to tolerate the drug regimens.

Patient Recruitment Status

Ongoing. Recruitment began in December 1992.

Current Status of Study

Ongoing.

Results

None to date.

Publications

Foscarnet-Ganciclovir Cytomegalovirus Retinitis Trial

Studies of Ocular Complications of AIDS (SOCA) Research Group in collaboration with the AIDS Clinical Trials Group (ACTG): Studies of Ocular Complications of AIDS Foscarnet-Ganciclovir Cytomegalovirus Retinitis Trial: (1) rationale, design, and methods. Controlled Clin Trials 1992; 13:22–39.

Studies of Ocular Complications of AIDS Research Group, in collaboration with the AIDS Clinical Trials Group: Mortality in patients with the acquired immunodeficiency syndrome treated with either foscarnet or ganciclovir for cytomegalovirus retinitis. N Engl J Med 1992;326:213–220.

CMV Retinitis Retreatment Trial

None.

Clinical Centers

California

Gary N. Holland, M.D.
Jules Stein Eye Institute
University of California, Los Angeles
100 Stein Plaza
Los Angeles, California 90024-7003
Telephone: (310) 825-9508

William R. Freeman, M.D.
Shiley Eye Center, 0946
University of California, San Diego
La Jolla, California 92093-0946
Telephone: (619) 534-3513

James O'Donnell, M.D.
Beckman Vision Center
University of California, San Francisco
Box 0730, Room K-301
10 Kirkham Street
San Francisco, California 94143
Telephone: (415) 476-1921

Florida

Janet Davis, M.D.
Bascom Palmer Eye Institute
University of Miami
900 N.W. 17th Street
Miami, Florida 33136
Telephone: (305) 326-4377

Illinois

David Weinberg, M.D.
Department of Ophthalmology

Northwestern University
222 East Superior Street
Chicago, Illinois 60611
Telephone: (312) 908-8040

Louisiana

Bruce A. Barron, M.D.
LSU Eye Center
Louisiana State University Medical Center
2020 Gravier Street, Suite B
New Orleans, Louisiana 70112
Telephone: (504) 568-6700 ext.307

Maryland

Douglas A. Jabs, M.D.
Wilmer Ophthalmological Institute
The Johns Hopkins Medical Institutions
Maumenee 119
600 North Wolfe Street
Baltimore, Maryland 21287-9217
Telephone: (410) 955-2966

New York

Murk-Hein Heinemann, M.D.
Department of Ophthalmology
Memorial Sloan-Kettering Cancer Center
1275 York Avenue, Suite A325
New York, New York 10021
Telephone: (212) 639-7237

Alan Friedman, M.D.
Department of Ophthalmology
Mount Sinai School of Medicine
Box 1183
One Gustave L. Levy Place
New York, New York 10029-4574
Telephone: (212) 241-6241

Dorothy Friedberg, M.D.
Department of Ophthalmology
New York University Medical Center
310 Lexington Avenue
New York, New York 10016
Telephone: (212) 687-0265

Texas

Richard Alan Lewis, M.D., M.S.
Cullen Eye Institute
Baylor College of Medicine
6501 Fannin Street, NC-200
Houston, Texas 77030
Telephone: (713) 798-4100

Resource Centers

Chairman's Office

Douglas A. Jabs, M.D.
Wilmer Ophthalmological Institute
The Johns Hopkins University and Hospital
550 North Broadway, Suite 700
Baltimore, Maryland 21205
Telephone: (410) 955-1966

Coordinating Center

Curtis L. Meinert, Ph.D.
Department of Epidemiology
School of Hygiene and Public Health
The Johns Hopkins University
615 North Wolfe Street, Room 5010
Baltimore, Maryland 21205
Telephone: (410) 955-8198

Fundus Photograph Reading Center

Matthew D. Davis, M.D.
Department of Ophthalmology
University of Wisconsin
610 North Walnut Street, Room 417
Madison, Wisconsin 53705-5240
Telephone: (608) 263-6071

Drug Distribution Center

Gary Stewart, M.S., R.Ph.
Ogden Bioservices Corporation
625 C Lofstrand Lane
Rockville, Maryland 20850
Telephone: (301) 762-0069

NEI Representative

Richard L. Mowery, Ph.D.
National Eye Institute
Executive Plaza South, Suite 350
6120 Executive Boulevard
Rockville, Maryland 20892
Telephone: (301) 496-5983

Policy and Data Monitoring Board

Byron William Brown, Jr., Ph.D., Chair
Stanford University
Stanford, CA

Brian P. Conway, M.D.
University of Virginia
Charlottesville, VA

James Grizzle, Ph.D.
Fred Hutchinson Cancer Research Center
Seattle, WA

Robert B. Nussenblatt, M.D.
National Eye Institute
Bethesda, MD

John Phair, M.D.
Northwestern University Medical School
Chicago, IL

Harmon Smith, Ph.D.
Duke University
Durham, NC

Richard J. Whitley, M.D.
University of Alabama at Birmingham
Birmingham, AL

Ex Officio Members

Matthew D. Davis, M.D.
University of Wisconsin
Madison, WI

Douglas A. Jabs, M.D.
Johns Hopkins University
Baltimore, MD

Joyce Korvick, M.D.
National Institute of Allergy and Infectious
   Diseases
Bethesda, MD

Curtis L. Meinert, Ph.D.
Johns Hopkins University
Baltimore, MD

Richard L. Mowery, Ph.D.
National Eye Institute
Bethesda, MD

James Tonascia, Ph.D.
Johns Hopkins University
Baltimore, MD

THE SILICONE STUDY

Study Chairman: Stephen J. Ryan, M.D.

Institutions: 13 Clinical Centers
3 Resource Centers

Purpose

- To compare, through a randomized, multicenter surgical trial, the postoperative tamponade effectiveness of intraocular silicone oil with that of an intraocular long-acting gas [initially sulfur hexafluoride (SF_6), later perfluoropropane (C_3F_8)] for the management of retinal detachment complicated by proliferative vitreoretinopathy (PVR) using vitrectomy and associated techniques.
- To evaluate the ocular complications that result from the use of silicone oil and gas.

Background

The treatment of retinal detachment complicated by PVR remains controversial. Although some cases are managed successfully by pars plana vitrectomy and with temporary tamponade provided by intraocular gas, others eventually redetach with this technique. Preliminary reports indicate that prolonged tamponade with liquid silicone results in improved anatomical success, but the eventual visual outcome may be prejudiced by silicone-related complications, particularly glaucoma and keratopathy. The addition to vitrectomy surgery of hydraulic reattachment by simultaneous fluid/gas exchange has proved to be an important development. Although complications are few with these procedures, subsequent redetachment is frequent.

Description

The Silicone Study is a randomized trial to investigate the relative merits of silicone oil or gas as tamponade modalities. All study patients undergo vitrectomy and are randomized intraoperatively to either silicone oil or gas. Two groups of eyes are entered into the study: eyes that have not had a prior vitrectomy (Group 1) and those that have undergone previous vitrectomy outside the study (Group 2).

A critical element in the study is a standardized surgical procedure for PVR. This surgical procedure, intended to relieve retinal traction by utilizing vitrectomy techniques, is followed by assessment of the relief provided by an intraocular air tamponade. The eye is randomized to silicone oil or gas only after completion of the entire surgical procedure in order to eliminate investigator bias that might develop through knowledge of the treatment modality. Patients are examined 5 to 14 days following the randomization and again at 1, 3, 6, 12, 18, 24, and 36 months after that date. Repeated surgery is permitted for either treatment modality. The Fundus Photograph Reading Center staff process and analyze photographs taken at all of the clinics, grade the preoperative severity of PVR on the basis of baseline visit photographs, and confirm the macular status at followup visits.

Endpoints of the study are visual acuity of 5/200 or greater and macular reattachment for 6 months following the final surgical procedure. The successful outcomes and complication rates of the two modalities will be compared.

Patient Eligibility

Eligibility criteria include, but was not limited to, PVR of Grade C-3 or greater, according to the Retina Society Classification, and visual acuity of light perception or better.

Patient Recruitment Status

Recruitment began on September 1, 1985, and was completed June 30, 1991. A total of 151 eyes were randomized to receive either SF_6 gas or silicone oil (113 in Group 1 and 38 in Group 2). Four hundred and four eyes were randomized to receive either C_3F_8 gas or silicone oil (232 and 172 in Groups 1 and 2, respectively).

Current Status of Study

Ongoing. Recruitment and 6-month followup is complete for 555 patients. Analyses comparing the results of each of the two gases to silicone oil are complete.

Continued study of patients with less than 36 months followup is underway to enable more valid comparisons of the long-term effects of silicone oil and C_3F_8 gas. In addition, those eyes with attached maculas will be studied for an additional 2 years to compare the rates of long-term visual loss and/or ocular complications in eyes from which silicone oil has been removed to those eyes permanently filled with silicone oil or treated with long-acting gas.

Results

Because C_3F_8 gas replaced the initially used SF_6 gas, we report two separate sets of results: one comparing SF6 gas to silicone oil used and one comparing C_3F_8 gas to silicone oil used during the period C_3F_8 gas was used.

Silicone oil was found to be superior to SF_6 gas in achieving functional visual acuity ($\geq 5/200$) and retinal reattachment in eyes with no previous vitrectomy. Complications, specifically hypotony and keratopathy, were more prevalent in the SF_6 gas-treated group. For eyes having undergone a previous vitrectomy, the sample size was too small to allow for a valid comparison of the two treatments.

The comparison of C_3F_8 gas to silicone oil suggests that C_3F_8 gas has a marginal advantage over silicone oil in achieving retinal reattachment in eyes with no previous vitrectomy. For this same group of eyes, there was no significant benefit with respect to visual results or complications. In the eyes having undergone a previous vitrectomy, there was no statistically significant differences in the anatomic or visual results between eyes randomized to C_3F_8 gas compared to silicone oil. However, the prevalence of hypotony was higher in eyes randomized to C_3F_8 gas.

Publications

Azen SP, DC, Barlow WE, Walonker AF, McCuen B, et al.: Methods, statistical features and baseline results of a standardized, multicentered ophthalmologic surgical trial: The Silicone Study. Controlled Gin Trials 1991;12:438–455.

Azen SP, Irvine AR, Davis MD, Stern WH, Lonn L, Hilton G, Schwartz A, Boone DC, Quillen-Thomas B, Lyons M, Lean J, Silicone Study Group: The validity and reliability of photographic documentation of proliferated vitreoretinopathy. Ophthalmology 1989;96:352–357.

Barlow WE, Azen SP: The effect of unscheduled crossovers on the power of a clinical trial. Controlled Clin Trials 1990; 11:314–326.

Glaser BM: Silicone Study Group: Silicone oil for proliferative vitreoretinopathy: Does it help or hinder? Arch Ophthalmol 1988;106:323–324.

Irvine AR: Photographic documentation and grading of PVR, in Freeman HM, Tolentino Fl (eds.): Proliferative Vitreoretinopathy, New York, Springer-Verlag, 1989;105–09.

Lean JS: Changing attitudes in United States to use of intravitreal silicone. Jpn J Ophthalmol 1987;31:132–139.

Lean JS, Stern WH, Irvine AR, Azen SP: Silicone Study Group: The Silicone Study classification of proliferative vitreoretinopathy. Ophthalmology 1989;96:765–771.

Stern WH, Lean JS: Silicone Study Group: Intraocular silicone oil versus gas in the management of proliferative vitreoretinopathy (PVR): A multicenter clinical study. In Freeman HM, Tolentino FL (eds.): Proliferative Vitreoretinopathy, New York, Springer-Verlag, 1989.

The Silicone Study Group: Proliferative vitreoretinopathy. Am J Ophthalmol 1985;99:593–595.

The Silicone Study Group: Vitrectomy with silicone oil or sulfur hexafluoride gas in eyes with severe proliferative vitreoretinopathy: Results of a randomized clinical trial-Silicone Study Report No.1. Arch Ophthalmol 1992;110: 770–779.

The Silicone Study Group: Vitrectomy with silicone oil or perfluoropropane gas in eyes with severe proliferative vitreoretinopathy: Results of a randomized clinical trial-Silicone Study Report No. 2. Arch Ophthalmol 1992;110: 780–792.

Clinical Centers

California

Allan E. Kreiger, M.D.
Doris Stein Eye Research Center
Jules Stein Eye Institute
UCLA School of Medicine
200 Stein Plaza, Retina Division
Los Angeles, California 90024-7007
Telephone: (213) 825-5477

John S. Lean, M.D.
1401 N. Tustin Avenue, Suite 220
Santa Ana, California 92701
Telephone: (714) 543-6020

Walter H. Stern, M.D.
Department of Ophthalmology
Beckman Vision Center, K-301
UCSF Medical Center
mailing address:
50 South San Mateo Drive, Suite 125
San Mateo, California 94401
Telephone: (415) 340-4111, (415) 969-7997

Florida

Harry Flynn, M.D.
Bascom Palmer Eye Institute
University of Miami School of Medicine
900 N.W. 17th Street
Miami, Florida 33136
Telephone: (305) 326-6350

Georgia

Thomas M. Aaberg M.D.
Department of Ophthalmology
Emory University School of Medicine
1327 Clifton Road, N.E.
Atlanta, Georgia 30322
Telephone: (404) 321-0111 x3710

Kentucky

Charles C. Barr, M.D.
Kentucky Retina Group
Kentucky Lions Eye Research Institute
University of Louisville School of Medicine
301 East Muhammad Ali Boulevard
Louisville, Kentucky 40202
Telephone: (502) 588-5466

Massachusetts

H. MacKenzie Freeman, M.D.
Retina Associates
100 Charles River Plaza
Cambridge Street

Boston, Massachusetts 02114
Telephone: (617) 523-7810

Michigan

Gary W. Abrams, M.D.
Morton S. Cox, M.D.
Associated Retinal Consultants
William Beaumont Medical Building,
Suite 632
3535 West Thirteen Mile Road
Royal Oak, Michigan 48072
Telephone: (313) 288-2280

Minnesota

Robert C. Ramsay, M.D.
Department of Ophthalmology
University of Minnesota
Mayo Memorial Building, Box 493516
Delaware Street, S.E.
Minneapolis, Minnesota 55455
Telephone: (612) 625-4400

North Carolina

Brooks W. McCuen, M.D.
Department of Ophthalmology
Duke University Medical Center
Box 3802
Durham, North Carolina 27710
Telephone: (919) 684-6749

Texas

William L. Hutton, M.D.
Texas Retina Associates
7150 Greenville Avenue, #400
Dallas, Texas 75231
Telephone: (214) 692-4941

Resource Centers

Chairman's Office

Stephen J. Ryan, M.D.
Estelle Doheny Eye Institute

USC School of Medicine
1355 San Pablo Avenue
Los Angeles, California 90033
Telephone: (213) 342-6444

Coordinating Center

Stanley P. Azen, Ph.D.
Division of Biometry
Department of Preventive Medicine
USC School of Medicine
1420 San Pablo Street, PMB B-101
Los Angeles, California 90033
Telephone: (213) 342-1810

Fundus Photograph Reading Center

Alexander R. Irvine, M.D.
UCSF Medical Center
400 Parnassus Avenue
San Francisco, California 94143
Telephone: (415) 476-4142

NEI Representative

Richard L. Mowery, Ph.D.
National Eye Institute
Executive Plaza South, Suite 350
6120 Executive Boulevard
Rockville, Maryland 20892
Telephone: (301) 496-5983

Data and Safety Monitoring Committee

Argye Hillis, Ph.D., Chair
Scott & White Hospital
Temple, TX

A.A. Afifi, Ph.D.
University of California
Los Angeles, CA

Daniel Finkelstein, M.D.
Johns Hopkins University
Baltimore, MD

Edward B. McLean, M.D.
Ophthalmic Consultants Northwest
Seattle, WA

TREATMENT OF ENDOGENOUS INTERMEDIATE AND POSTERIOR UVEITIS BY ORAL TOLERIZATION TO RETINAL S-ANTIGEN

Principal Investigator: Robert B. Nussenblatt, M.D.

Institution: 1 Clinical Center–NIH

Purpose

To evaluate the effectiveness of the oral administration of retinal S-Antigen and/or a crude retinal mixture in the induction of tolerance to retinal S-Antigen in endogenous uveitis patients who are in need of systemic immunotherapy.

Background

Uveitis, an intraocular inflammatory disease, is the cause of about 10 percent of visual impairment in the United States. Treatment for severe, sight-threatening uveitis has primarily involved the use of pharmacologic substances that have a non-specific effect on the immune response. Recent studies have investigated the effect of cyclosporine, which has a predominantly anti-T cell mode of action, on the immune response without respect to the specific antigen evoking the response. All of the treatments used to date are effective to some degree, but all have inherent serious side effects. Therefore, one of the goals of immunotherapy of sight-threatening endogenous uveitis is to find an immunospecific and relatively non-toxic therapy that can be administered early in the course of the disease. An animal model for human uveitis, known as experimental autoimmune uveitis, has been developed by immunization of the animal with S-Antigen, a uveitagenic retinal protein. It was determined that feeding S-Antigen to these animals prevented the development of experimental autoimmune uveitis. Suppressor cells from fed animals could be transferred to naive hosts and the disease would be suppressed in them as well. Of interest was the observation that not all fragments of the S-Antigen were capable of preventing the disease when given orally, suggesting that certain parts of the molecule were more important than others in the induction of tolerance.

Because of the remarkable effect of S-Antigen feeding in animals, a pilot study in people with uveitis was undertaken after Food and Drug Administration approval. One male and one female patient were selected using two major criteria. The first was the patients had received long-term treatment for their uveitis with systemic medication, and when they were weaned from the medication they suffered a recurrence of the disease. The second was that their lymphocytes, when cultured *in vitro,* demonstrated an anamnestic (i.e., memory) response to the retinal S-Antigen. The patients were fed the retinal S-Antigen for 3 weeks with no change in the dose of their regular medication. After this time, the patients were slowly weaned off their immunosuppressive medications and continued to be fed the S-Antigen. It was noted that these patients could be taken off their regular medications and maintain good vision. Because of these initial positive results, a masked randomized trial was designed to determine whether or not oral tolerization could be applied to uveitis.

Description

A randomized, double-masked study has been designed to evaluate the efficacy and safety of oral tolerization of ocular antigens in the treatment of uveitis patients.

Patients will be randomized to one of three arms of the study: the retinal S-Antigen, a retinal mixture containing all of the soluble retinal components, or placebo. Patients will be treated for 3 weeks with the masked formulation, and at the end of the 3-week period their regular immuno-suppressive medication will be slowly reduced for the next 2 months. The intent is to take the patients completely off their regular medication. Primary end points include recurrence of disease as well as disease activity assessed by clinical examination. A secondary goal will be to evaluate the potential medication sparing effect of oral tolerization.

A total of 45 patients will be recruited for the study. Patients will be seen at baseline and weeks 3, 6, 8, 12, and 26 after enrollment into the study.

Patient Eligibility

Males and females of all ages who have bilateral sight-threatening uveitis and are taking systemic immune suppressive medication to maintain good visual acuity. Patients will have blood drawn (about 20–25 cc) to test for an in *vitro* proliferative response to the retinal S-Antigen, which is also required for entry into the study. Exclusion criteria include old disease that no longer requires active immuno-suppression, and possible ocular surgery during the period of the study.

Patient Recruitment Status

Ongoing. Recruitment began November 1992.

Current Status of Study

Ongoing.

Results

None to date.

Publications

Nussenblatt RB, Caspi R, Mahdi R, Chan CC, Roberge F, Lider O, and Weiner HL: Inhibition of S-Antigen induced experimental autoimmune uveoretinitis by oral induction of tolerance with S-Antigen. J Immunol 1990;144:1689–1695.

Clinical Center

Robert B. Nussenblatt, M.D.
National Eye Institute
National Institutes of Health
Warren Grant Magnuson Clinical Center
Building 10, Room 10N202
Bethesda, Maryland 20892
Telephone: (301) 496-3123

Index

Note: Page numbers followed by *t* and *f* indicate tables and figures, respectively.